COLOUR GUI

PICTURE TES

Ophthalmology

Jack J. Kanski MD MS FRCS FRCOphth

Consultant Ophthalmic Surgeon
Prince Charles Eye Unit
King Edward VII Hospital
Windsor

Ken K. Nischal FRCOphth

Senior House Officer
Prince Charles Eye Unit
King Edward VII Hospital
Windsor

SECOND EDITION

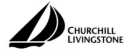

CHURCHILL
LIVINGSTONE

EDINBURGH LONDON MADRID MELBOURNE NEW YORK AND TOKYO 1997

CHURCHILL LIVINGSTONE
An imprint of Harcourt Publishers Limited

First edition 1994
Second edition 1997
Reprinted 2000, 2002

ISBN 0-443-06037-1

British Library Cataloguing in Publication Data
A catalogue record for this book is available from the British
Library.

Library of Congress Cataloging in Publication Data
A catalog record for this book is available from the Library
of Congress.

For Churchill Livingstone

Publisher
Michael Parkinson
Project Editor
Jim Killgore
Production
Nancy Arnott
Design direction
Erik Bigland

The
publisher's
policy is to use
**paper manufactured
from sustainable forests**

Printed in China by RDC Group Limited
P/03

Preface

This book is primarily intended for resident ophthalmologists both as a learning tool and a self-assessment guide. Although the bulk of the factual knowledge lies in the answer section there are important epidemiological facts in each question stem. We hope that the style of questions and answers will be particularly helpful for the viva voce and short cases presentations in post-graduate examinations.

Windsor   J.J.K.
1994   K.K.N.

Acknowledgements

We are very grateful to Mr. P. Watts for providing us with some of the questions and slides. We would also like to thank A. Nischal in helping with the manuscript and a special thanks, on behalf of K.K.N., to P.R. Nischal for her support and encouragement.

The following colleagues and Eye Departments very kindly provided us with slides: Prof. A. Bird (Fig. 26); Mr. P. Watson (Fig. 160); Mr. M. Sanders (Fig. 141); Prof. B. Jay (Figs 4 and 146); Mr. T. Ffytche (Fig. 5); Mr. D. Taylor (Fig. 18); Mr. K. Jordan (Fig. 39); Mr. R. Collin (Fig. 107); Mr. J. Bell (Fig. 174); and Western Ophthalmic Hospital (Figs 37, 50, 82, 91, 95, 112 & 150).

Test answers begin on page 101.
Index—page 163.

Questions

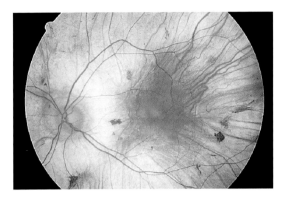

1. This is the fundus of a 30-year-old man who has had defective night vision since the age of 7 years. The fellow eye has a similar appearance.

a. What is the diagnosis and mode of inheritance?
b. What biochemical abnormality may be present?
c. What may be the appearance of his mother's fundus?

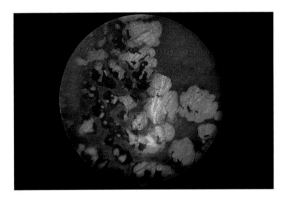

2. This is the fundus of a 20-year-old female who developed defective night vision at the age of 9 years. The fellow eye has a similar appearance.

a. What is the diagnosis?
b. What is the metabolic error in this condition?
c. What is the mode of inheritance?
d. What other ocular lesions may be present?

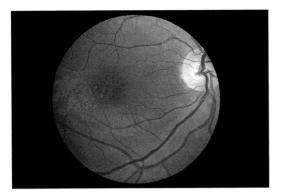

3. This is the fundus of an 18-year-old male who failed his driving test because his visual acuity was 6/18. The other eye has a similar appearance.

a. What is the diagnosis?
b. What is the mode of inheritance?
c. What other fundus lesions may be present?
d. What are the systemic associations?

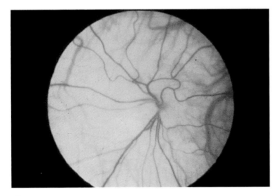

4. This is the fundus of a 10-year-old boy with very pale skin and pendular nystagmus.

a. What are the signs?
b. What is the diagnosis?
c. What other ocular and neurological abnormalities may be present?
d. Why could this child's life be in danger?

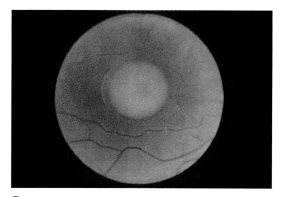

5. This is the fundus of a 15-year-old boy with a visual acuity of 6/9 in both eyes and a severely reduced electro-oculogram. The fellow eye has a similar appearance.

a. What is the diagnosis?
b. What is the mode of inheritance?
c. What are the five stages of this condition?
d. What is the long-term visual prognosis?

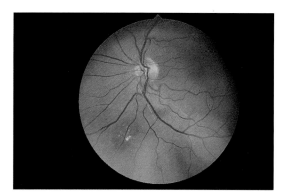

6. This asymptomatic lesion was discovered by chance during a routine fundus examination of a 35-year-old myopic female.

a. What is the diagnosis?
b. What may fundus fluorescein angiography show?
c. What percentage of these lesions are located posterior to the equator?
d. What complications may arise?

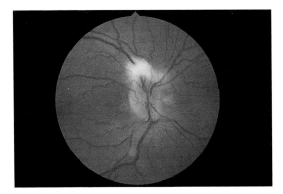

7. **This is the fundus of a 22-year-old male with headache who was thought to have papilloedema by his general practitioner.**

a. What is the diagnosis?
b. What is the mode of inheritance?
c. In what percentage of cases are both eyes affected?
d. What is the gender distribution?
e. In which way may vision be affected?

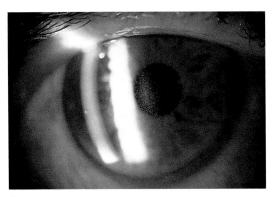

8. **This 35-year-old myopic man has raised intraocular pressures in both eyes.**

a. What are the signs?
b. What is the diagnosis?
c. What is the mode of inheritance of this condition?
d. What other anterior segment findings may be observed?

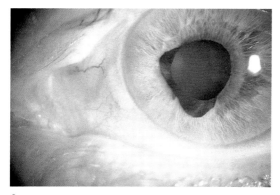

9. This 7-month-old girl was noted to have iris abnormality since birth.

a. What is the diagnosis?
b. What is the management?
c. What systemic disease may she have?

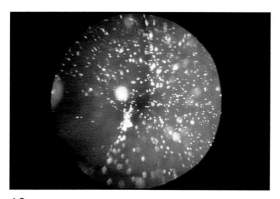

10. This is the vitreous of a 65-year-old female.

a. What is the diagnosis?
b. Is her visual acuity likely to be impaired?
c. What underlying systemic disease may she have?
d. What is the differential diagnosis?

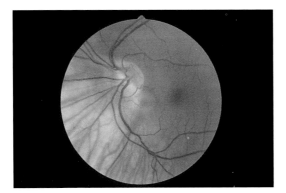

11. This is the fundus of a 40-year-old man with severe headache who was referred to a neurologist because he was found to have bilateral upper temporal visual field defects. The fellow eye has a similar appearance.

a. What is the fundus diagnosis?
b. What is the mode of inheritance?
c. What is the cause of his visual field defects?
d. Why does he have headache?

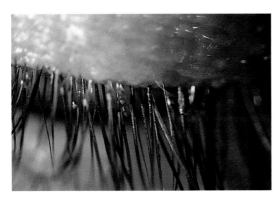

12. This child was sent to the ophthalmologist after a routine examination at school.

a. What is the diagnosis?
b. What is the treatment?
c. Where else in the body might this be found?

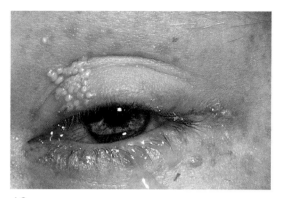

13. This patient was referred with a painful vesicular eruption on the right upper lid. Assuming no other lesions were found elsewhere:

a. Could this be shingles?
b. What is the most likely diagnosis?
c. Would you treat this with acyclovir cream or ointment, or both?

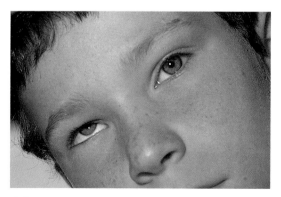

14. This 10-year-old boy sustained a closed head injury four days ago and developed vertical diplopia. He was found to have a right hypertropia which increased on head tilt to the right shoulder (as shown here).

a. What is the diagnosis?
b. What compensatory head posture may he adopt?
c. What surgical procedures may correct the defect?

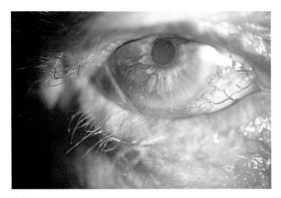

15. Three months ago this 74-year-old female developed severe blurring of vision in this eye. Three days ago the eye became very painful and the intraocular pressure was found to be 62 mmHg.

a. What does the picture show?
b. What is the likely cause of her visual loss three months ago?
c. Why is the intraocular pressure raised?
d. What other conditions may cause the same appearance?

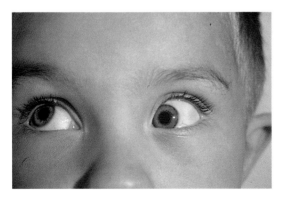

16. At the age of 3 years this child was found to be unable to dextro-elevate the left eye. There was also divergence in upgaze.

a. What is the probable diagnosis?
b. How many cases are bilateral?
c. What is the treatment?
d. Which conditions may cause a similar ocular motility defect?

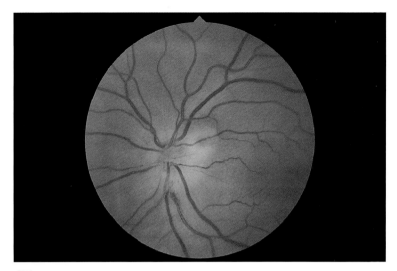

17. This is the fundus of an 81-year-old man who developed a sudden and profound loss of vision in this eye one day ago.

a. What is the probable diagnosis and pathogenesis?
b. What are the possible causes?
c. What investigations would be appropriate in this patient?

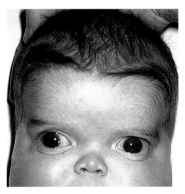

18. This child has bilateral primary congenital glaucoma.

a. What are the signs?
b. What is the mode of inheritance?
c. What may be seen on gonioscopy?
d. What is the initial treatment of most cases?
e. What are the main causes of visual impairment?

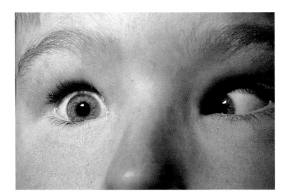

19. This 4-year-old girl is attempting to look to the right. The parents noticed that the right eye could move to the left but seemed to become smaller.

a. What is the likely diagnosis?
b. What percentage of cases are bilateral?
c. What systemic problems may she have?
d. When is surgical treatment appropriate?

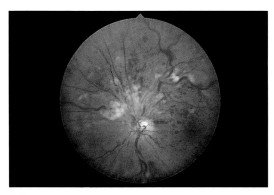

20. This is the fundus of a 65-year-old hypertensive who noticed that he had very poor vision on waking up in the morning three days ago.

a. What is the diagnosis?
b. What is the main classification of this condition?
c. What are possible underlying causes?

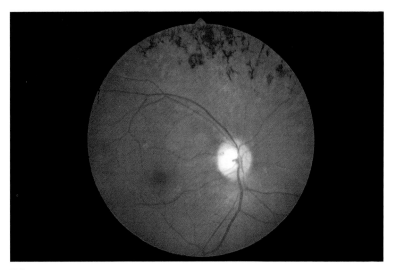

21. This is the fundus of a patient with typical retinitis pigmentosa.

a. What are the main atypical forms?
b. What macular lesions may the patient have?
c. What associated ocular lesions may be present?

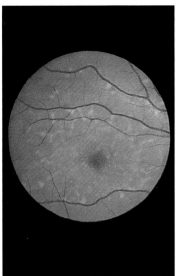

22. This is the fundus of a 15-year-old boy who developed mild visual impairment 6 years ago.

a. What is the likely diagnosis?
b. What is the usual mode of inheritance?
c. What are the four main patterns of this disorder?
d. What other ocular lesions may be present?

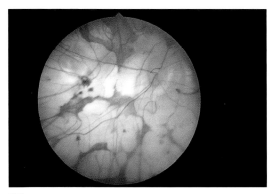

23. This is the fundus of a very high myope with a visual acuity of 6/60.

a. What are lacquer cracks?
b. What types of maculopathy may occur in this eye?
c. What are other potential ocular complications?
d. What are the main systemic associations?

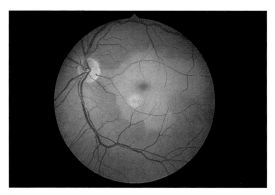

24. This is the fundus of a 66-year-old man who noted a sudden and profound loss of central vision in this eye one day ago.

a. What is the diagnosis?
b. What is the likely cause?
c. Why does the fovea appear red?

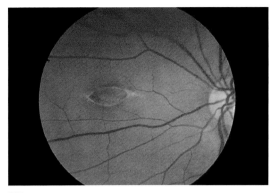

25. This is the fundus of a 25-year-old man whose brother died at the age of 36 years from carcinoma of the colon.

a. What is the fundus diagnosis?
b. What is the probable systemic diagnosis?
c. What is the mode of inheritance?
d. How should this patient be managed?

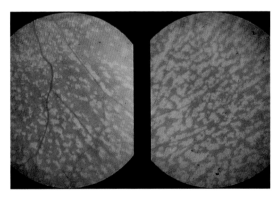

26. This 24-year-old female has been night blind from birth but has normal visual acuity in both eyes.

a. What is the likely diagnosis?
b. What is the mode of inheritance?
c. What is the visual prognosis?
d. What is the differential diagnosis?

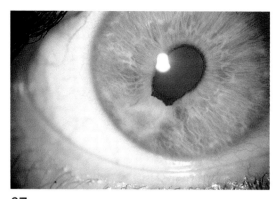

27. This lesion has doubled in size during the last 2 years.

a. What is the likely diagnosis?
b. What is the differential diagnosis?
c. What is the prognosis?
d. What are the treatment options?

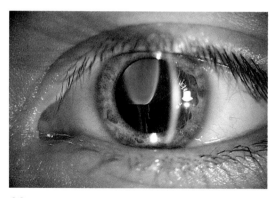

28. This 7-year-old girl was found to have bilateral ectopia lentis.

a. What is ectopia lentis?
b. What is the difference between luxation and subluxation?
c. Which syndromes are associated with ectopia lentis?
d. Which metabolic disorders are associated with ectopia lentis?

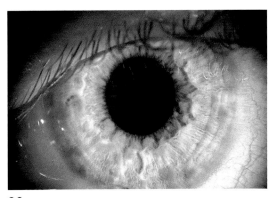

29. These iris lesions were discovered in a 17-year-old male who was found to have slight proptosis and mild optic atrophy in the other eye.

a. What are the iris lesions?
b. What is their pathology?
c. What is the probable underlying systemic disorder?
d. What could be the cause of the signs in his other eye?
e. What other ophthalmic lesions may be present?

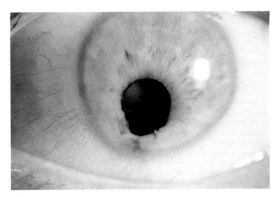

30. This abnormality has been present from birth. The other eye has a similar appearance.

a. What is the diagnosis?
b. What is the mode of inheritance?
c. What is the pathogenesis?
d. What other ocular lesions may be present?
e. What are possible systemic associations?

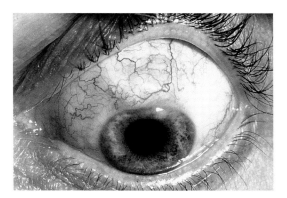

31. This 65-year-old man had a trabeculectomy for uncontrolled primary open-angle glaucoma. Four weeks later the intraocular pressure is 35 mmHg.

a. What is the diagnosis?
b. What factors may contribute to initial failure of filtration?
c. How may the risks of failed filtration be reduced?

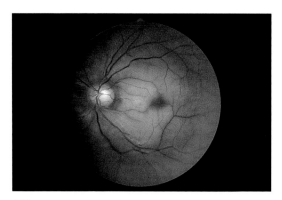

32. This 16-year-old boy presented to casualty 24 hours after being hit on the eye by a football.

a. What is the diagnosis?
b. What is the natural history of this condition?
c. What other posterior segment complications may he develop?

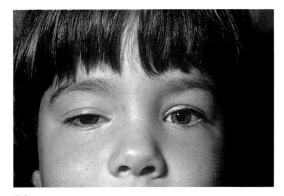

33. This 5-year-old girl has a right congenital ptosis with 8 mm of levator function.

a. Clinically how do you grade the severity of ptosis?
b. How do you assess levator function?
c. What is the optimal age to correct congenital ptosis?
d. What operation would you perform?

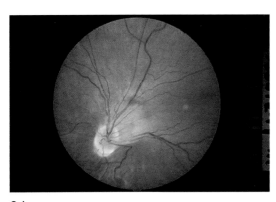

34. This is the fundus of a 6-year-old boy with retinopathy of prematurity.

a. What does the fundus show?
b. What is threshold disease?
c. How should neonates at risk be screened?

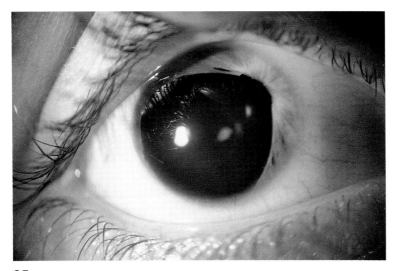

35. This is the eye of a 35-year-old man with congenital nystagmus and a visual acuity of 3/60. The fellow eye has a similar appearance.

a. What is the diagnosis?
b. What are the phenotypes of this condition?
c. What are the modes of inheritance?
d. What other ocular defects may be present?

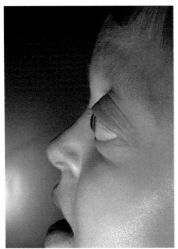

36. This is the appearance of a 7-year-old boy with 3/60 visual acuity in both eyes.

a. What is the diagnosis?
b. What are the possible causes of poor vision in this condition?
c. What other ocular problems may he have?
d. Is this patient likely to be mentally retarded?

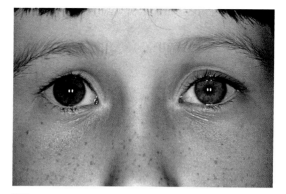

37. This 10-year-old girl has heterochromia iridis.

a. What other signs are present?
b. What are the main congenital causes of heterochromia iridis?
c. What are acquired causes of heterochromia?

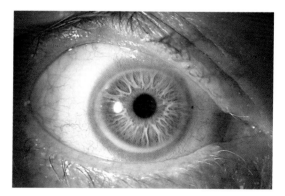

38. This 42-year-old man presented with two episodes of temporary loss of vision in his right eye lasting between 15 and 20 minutes.

a. What is this symptom called?
b. What is the condition shown above?
c. Classify the hyperlipidaemias.
d. How else can hyperlipidaemias affect the eye?

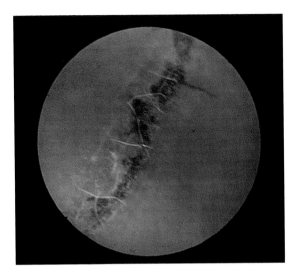

39. This is the peripheral retina of a 36-year-old moderate myope who developed a retinal detachment in his fellow eye.

a. What is the diagnosis?
b. What are the systemic associations?
c. What are the indications for prophylactic treatment?
d. What is the most common complication of prophylactic treatment?

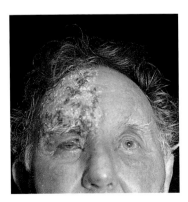

40. This man presented 5 days after the onset of the rash with blurred vision in the ipsilateral eye.

a. What is the cause of his rash?
b. How would you treat the rash?
c. What could be the cause of his blurred vision?
d. What neurological complications may he develop?

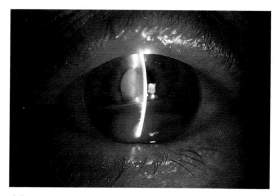

41. **This man was hit on the eye by a tennis ball one hour ago.**

a. What is the diagnosis?
b. What other anterior segment injuries may be present?
c. What are the current potential vision-threatening complications?
d. What is your management?

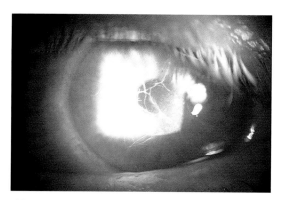

42. **This is the cornea of a 35-year-old man who developed recurrent corneal erosions at the age of 8 years.**

a. What is the diagnosis?
b. What is the mode of inheritance?
c. What is the composition of the material?
d. What are the staining properties of this material?
e. What systemic disease may this man have?

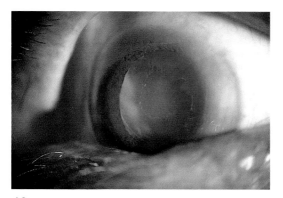

43. This 60-year-old female patient was found to have raised intraocular pressure and glaucomatous cupping in this eye.

a. What is the diagnosis?
b. What is the risk of glaucoma in the fellow eye?
c. What is the origin of the material seen on the lens?
d. What is Sampaolesi's line?
e. What problems might be encountered if this patient required cataract extraction?

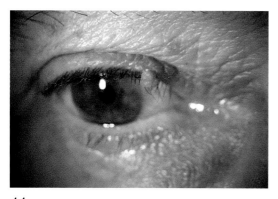

44. This benign tumour has been present for 7 years in a 56-year-old female.

a. What is the probable diagnosis?
b. How should it be removed?
c. What are the histological features?
d. What other benign (not premalignant) tumours may occur on the eyelids?

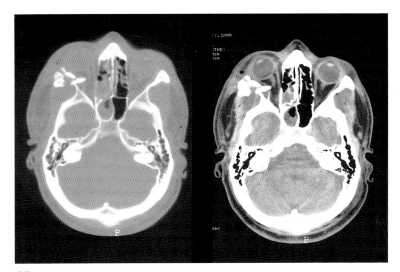

45. This is a CT scan of a patient who was assaulted and knocked unconscious. He was found to have a subconjunctival haemorrhage the posterior margin of which could not be visualized and also a Battle sign.

a. What may be the significance of the subconjunctival haemorrhage?
b. What is the Battle sign?
c. What might be his pupillary reactions?

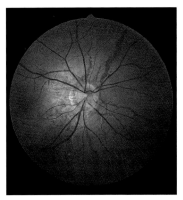

46. This is the fundus of a 26-year-old female who presented to casualty with a severe upper gastrointestinal bleed. The visual acuity in her other eye has been impaired for the last 3 years.

a. What is the fundus diagnosis?
b. What may be the cause of the poor vision in the other eye?
c. What could be the cause of her gastrointestinal haemorrhage?
d. What other systemic conditions may have similar fundus changes?

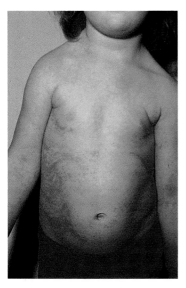

47. This young girl was found to have leukocoria at the age of 9 months.

a. What is the systemic diagnosis?
b. What is the mode of inheritance?
c. What are the systemic manifestations?
d. What is the likely cause of her leukocoria?

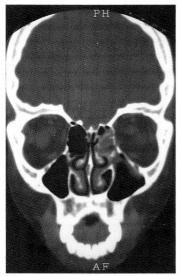

48. This is the CT scan of a patient who was hit on the eye with a fist during an assault.

a. What is the diagnosis?
b. What clinical signs may be present?
c. What is the initial treatment?
d. What are the main indications for surgical intervention?

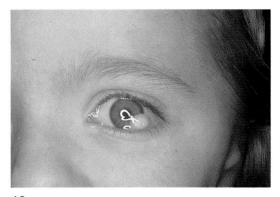

49. This girl is hard of hearing.

a. What is the ocular diagnosis?
b. What is the possible systemic diagnosis?
c. What other ocular abnormalities may she have?

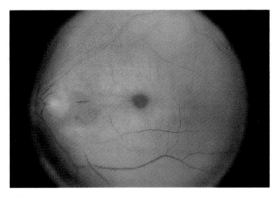

50. This is the fundus of a 60-year-old man with ischaemic heart disease who developed a sudden loss of vision 4 hours ago.

a. What is the diagnosis?
b. What is the immediate management?
c. What is the visual prognosis?
d. What are other vascular causes of sudden visual loss?

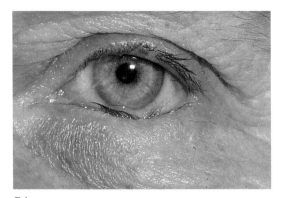

51. This patient complains of chronic unilateral ocular irritation.

a. What is the diagnosis?
b. How do you classify this condition?
c. Which surgical procedures may be used to correct the problem?

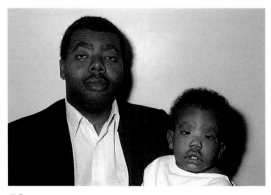

52. This is a father and his 3-year-old daughter.

- What is the diagnosis?
- What are the main clinical features?
- What is the treatment?

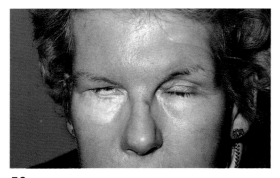

53. This lady has a right facial palsy and is trying to close her eyes.

a. What phenomenon is shown?
b. Is the absence of this phenomenon necessarily pathological?
c. What ocular complication may arise?
d. How may it be prevented?

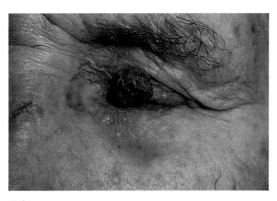

54. This is a very common skin lesion seen in the elderly.

a. Its main histological features are hyperkeratosis, acanthosis and papillomatosis. Define these terms.
b. What is the diagnosis?
c. Should the lesion be removed?
d. Name four premalignant eyelid lesions.

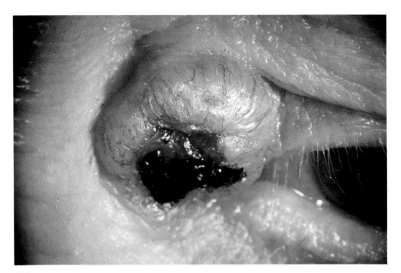

55. This lesion in a 70-year-old man has been growing slowly for the last 2 years.

a. What is the likely diagnosis?
b. What is the risk of metastasis?
c. If the patient was 25 years old which syndrome might he have?

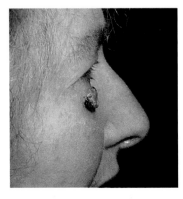

56. This lesion began to appear 6 weeks ago in a patient who had a renal transplant and was on immunosuppressives.

a. What is the likely diagnosis?
b. Is it associated with his systemic disease?
c. What is the natural history of the lesion?
d. What is the treatment?

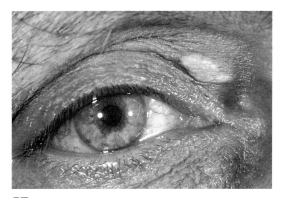

57. This 72-year-old lady has had this lesion for the last 12 years.

a. What is the diagnosis?
b. What are the risks of malignant transformation?
c. Are there any systemic associations?
d. Where else may similar lesions be found?

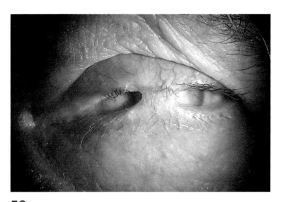

58. This 72-year-old lady had this procedure performed 3 months previously.

a. What was the procedure?
b. What are the main indications?
c. Describe an alternative method to achieve lid closure.

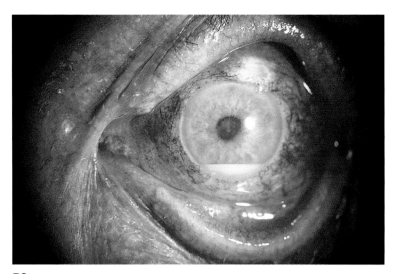

59. This patient had an uneventful trabeculectomy 4 weeks ago and now presents with a painful eye and blurred vision.

a. What is the diagnosis?
b. What are the predisposing factors?
c. What is the immediate management?

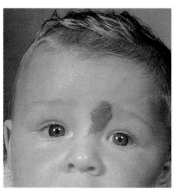

60. This lesion has been present since birth.

a. What is the diagnosis?
b. Is removal indicated?
c. What is the Kasabach–Merritt syndrome?

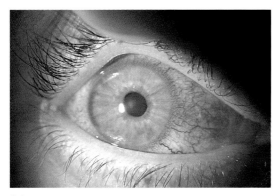

61. This 32-year-old man, with known ankylosing spondylitis, presents with a photophobic eye.

a. What is the diagnosis?
b. Why is the patient photophobic?
c. What is the visual prognosis?

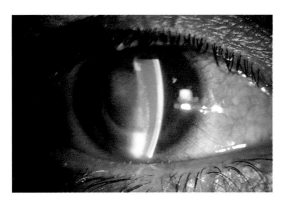

62. This patient with Reiter's syndrome has a very severe anterior uveitis with fibrin formation in the anterior chamber.

a. What is Reiter's syndrome?
b. How would you manage this patient?
c. What is the classic radiological finding in Reiter's syndrome?

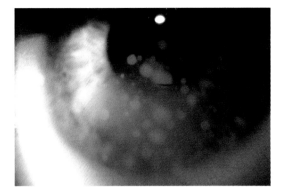

63. This patient has chronic anterior uveitis.

a. What are the signs?
b. What is the Ehrlich–Turk line?
c. What would be the pathological description of this type of intraocular inflammation?
d. What other anterior segment signs may be present?
e. What is the possible aetiology?

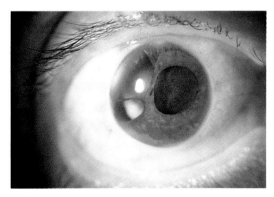

64. This is the eye of a 25-year-old male. The fellow eye has similar but less severe changes.

a. What is the diagnosis?
b. What is the mode of inheritance?
c. What ocular complications may be present?
d. Are there any systemic associations?

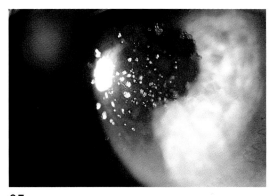

65. This is the cornea of a patient with irritable eyes.

a. What are the signs?
b. What is the composition of the lesions?
c. What are possible underlying causes?

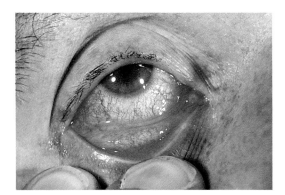

66. This patient has had bilateral sore and sticky eyes for 3 days.

a. What are the main types of infective conjunctivitis?
b. In order of preference what are your drugs of choice to treat bacterial conjunctivitis?
c. Which non-infectious systemic disorders may be associated with conjunctival inflammation?

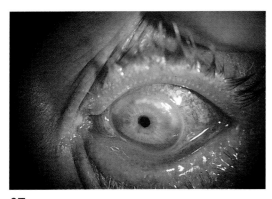

67. **This 50-year-old man with chronic staphylococcal blepharitis complained of a sore eye for 4 days.**

a. What are the signs?
b. What is the diagnosis?
c. Is the condition related to his blepharitis?
d. What is the treatment?

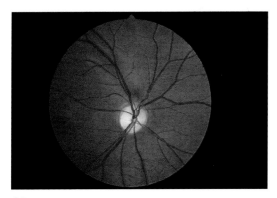

68. **This is the optic disc of a 32-year-old man who is thought to have inherited a predisposition to this condition. The fellow disc has a similar appearance.**

a. What is the ophthalmic diagnosis?
b. Which hereditary conditions may cause this condition?
c. What is the Foster–Kennedy syndrome?

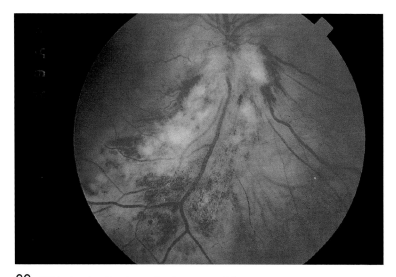

69. This is the fundus of a 35-year-old man on immunosuppressive therapy following a renal transplant.

a. What is the diagnosis?
b. Can this condition occur in healthy individuals?
c. What is the treatment?
d. What other fundus lesions may occur in immunocompromised individuals?

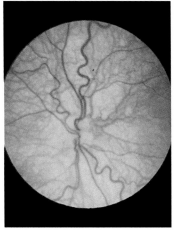

70. This is the fundus of an 8-year-old ataxic boy whose 'amblyopia' did not respond to occlusion.

a. What is the ocular diagnosis?
b. What is the mode of inheritance?
c. What could be the cause of his ataxia?
d. What other ocular anomalies may be present?

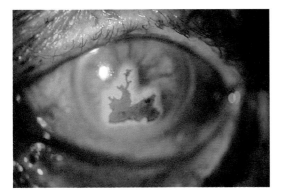

71. This patient's sore red eye has been treated with topical steroids for one week.

a. What is the diagnosis?
b. What is the treatment?
c. What might have happened had the patient presented one week later?

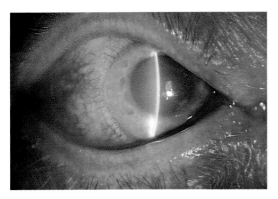

72. This is the eye of a patient with acute congestive primary angle-closure glaucoma with an intraocular pressure of 65 mmHg.

a. What is the treatment?
b. What is the classification of primary angle-closure glaucoma?
c. What are the mechanisms of chronic angle-closure glaucoma?

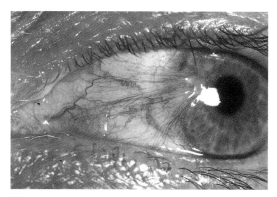

73. This 32-year-old Australian professional golfer noticed this lesion on his eye 3 years ago.

a. What is the diagnosis?
b. Does this condition have a racial predisposition?
c. What are the indications for surgical removal?
d. How can recurrence be prevented after excision?
e. What is the differential diagnosis?

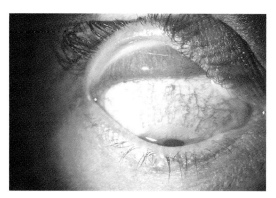

74. This is the eye of a 45-year-old female with a 2-year history of chronic bilateral non-specific ocular irritation associated with a slight mucoid discharge.

a. What is the probable diagnosis?
b. Would any serological test be appropriate?
c. What are the treatment options?

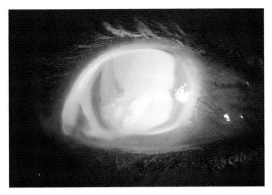

75. This diabetic was poked in the eye by his baby daughter.

a. What is the diagnosis?
b. Why is the lesion bright green?
c. What are the possible long-term complication?

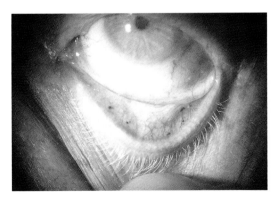

76. This is the inferior fornix of a 58-year-old man. He thinks the appearance of these lesions is related to the drops he takes for glaucoma.

a. Is he right?
b. If so should the drops be stopped?
c. Are the black deposits melanin?

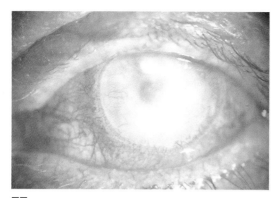

77. One week ago this 35-year-old patient developed pain and severe blurring of vision. On examination corneal sensation was reduced but there was no epithelial defect. There was no past history of trauma or contact lens wear.

a. What is the differential diagnosis?
b. What is the most likely diagnosis?
c. What is the treatment?

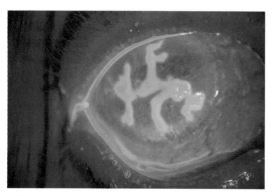

78. This 35-ear-old female noticed discomfort and blurred vision in this eye 10 days ago.

a. What is the diagnosis?
b. Which drugs can be used to treat this condition?
c. Which conditions can give rise to a similar appearance?

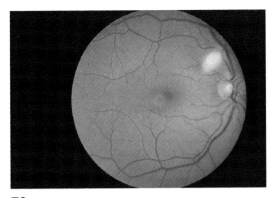

79. This is the fundus of a 45-year-old asymptomatic male.

a. What is the diagnosis?
b. What is the pathogenesis?
c. What are possible causes?

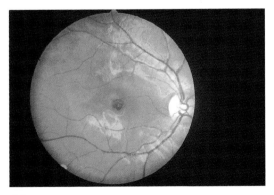

80. This emmetropic 70-year-old female noted blurred vision in her eye by chance when she covered the other eye.

a. What is the diagnosis?
b. What is the risk to the other eye?
c. What is the risk of retinal detachment?
d. What are other causes of a similar appearance?

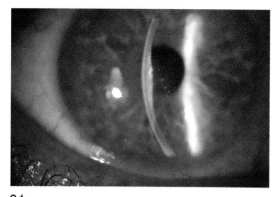

81. This 36-year-old lady presented with a painful eye and reduced visual acuity. On examination, the cornea was anaesthetic and showed the above signs.

a. Describe the signs.
b. What is the diagnosis?
c. What is a Wessley ring?

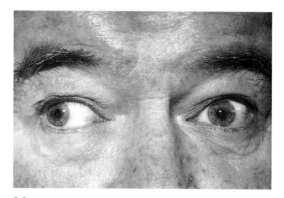

82. This patient with known multiple sclerosis developed diplopia 2 weeks ago which was worse on looking to the right.

a. What is the probable diagnosis?
b. What other ocular motility defects occur in multiple sclerosis?
c. What may MR of the brain show?

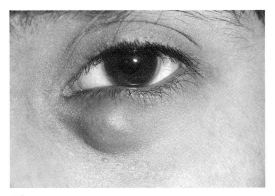

83. This 10-year-old child has had this painless lump in the lower eyelid for about 6 weeks.

a. What is the likely diagnosis?
b. Are there any predispositions?
c. What is the differential diagnosis?
d. What is the treatment?

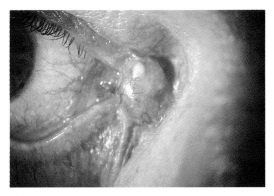

84. This asymptomatic translucent cyst has been present for over a year.

a. What is the likely diagnosis?
b. Are there any predispositions?
c. What is the differential diagnosis?
d. What is the treatment?

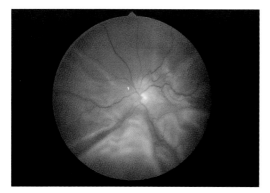

85. This picture shows a total retinal detachment.

a. What is a retinal detachment?
b. What are the main types of retinal detachment?
c. What are the signs of a long-standing rhegmatogenous retinal detachment?

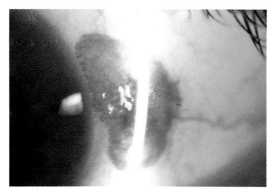

86. A 15-year-old boy has had this tumour for over 6 years. Recently it has been getting slightly larger and more pigmented.

a. What is the diagnosis?
b. What is the risk of malignant change?
c. What are the indications for surgical removal?
d. What are other benign tumours of the conjunctiva?

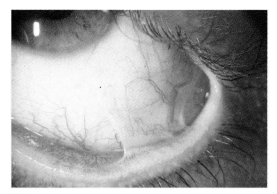

87. This is the conjunctiva of a patient with ocular cicatricial pemphigoid.

a. What are the signs?
b. What other ocular complications occur?
c. What other conditions may give rise to a similar appearance?

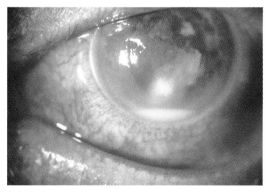

88. This patient has severe bacterial keratitis.

a. What are potential predisposing factors?
b. Which organisms are able to penetrate an intact corneal epithelium?
c. What is the immediate management?

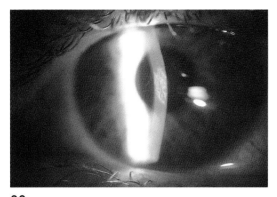

89. The visual acuity of this 24-year-old man could not be improved to better than 6/24 in the right eye and 6/18 in the left eye. Both eyes have the same condition.

a. What is the diagnosis?
b. Is corneal grafting appropriate in this patient?
c. What associated disorder may the patient have?

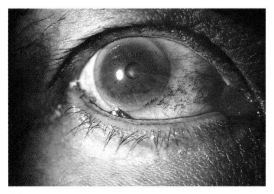

90. This is the eye of a 52-year-old female with sore eyes and seropositive rheumatoid arthritis following the instillation of rose bengal drops.

a. Why has rose bengal been used?
b. What is an abnormal Schirmer's test value?
c. What is an abnormal tear film break-up time?
d. What are the systemic associations in secondary Sjögren's syndrome?

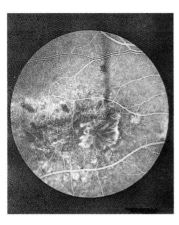

91. This is the fluorescein angiogram of a 72-year-old man who noticed metamorphopsia 10 days ago.

a. What is metamorphopsia?
b. What is the diagnosis?
c. What is the probable cause in this patient?
d. What are other important causes?

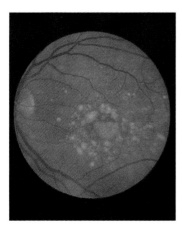

92. This is the fundus of a 66-year-old asymptomatic female who was thought to have background diabetic retinopathy by her optometrist.

a. What is the correct diagnosis?
b. How do you classify these retinal lesions?
c. What is their histology?
d. What is this patient's long-term visual prognosis?

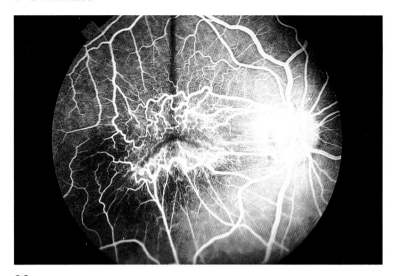

93. This is the fluorescein angiogram of a healthy 68-year-old man with no previous eye disease who developed severe metamorphopsia 6 months ago.

a. What is the diagnosis?
b. What is the probable cause in this patient?
c. What is the risk to the fellow eye?
d. What are other causes of this condition?

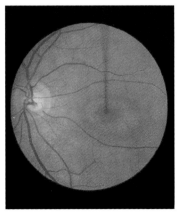

94. This is the fundus of a 35-year-old female on treatment for severe systemic lupus erythematosus.

a. What is the name given to this fundal appearance?
b. What is the probable cause in this patient?
c. What are other causes of a similar appearance?
d. What is the appearance on fluorescein angiography?

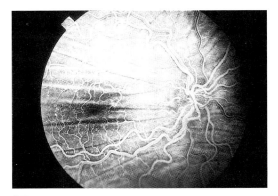

95. This is the fluorescein angiogram of a healthy hypermetropic 35-year-old man with normal corrected visual acuity.

a. What is the diagnosis?
b. What is the likely cause in this patient?
c. What are other causes?
d. How do you explain the angiographic features?

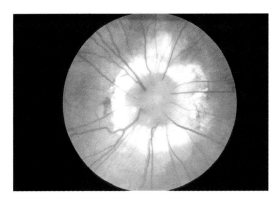

96. This is the fundus of a 6-year-old boy who was found to have defective vision on a routine school test.

a. What is the diagnosis?
b. What is the mode of inheritance?
c. Is this condition usually unilateral or bilateral?
d. What are possible systemic associations?

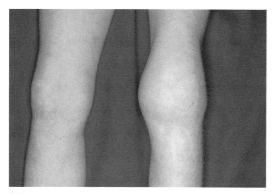

97. This is a 5-year-old girl with juvenile chronic arthritis.

a. What is the definition of juvenile chronic arthritis?
b. What are the main types?
c. What are the main risk factors for the development of ocular complications?
d. What is juvenile 'rheumatoid' arthritis?

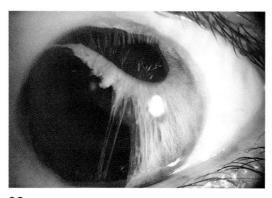

98. This is a glaucomatous eye in a 40-year-old female.

a. What is the diagnosis?
b. What is the mode of inheritance?
c. What are the gonioscopical findings?
d. What is the risk to the fellow eye?
e. What is the differential diagnosis?

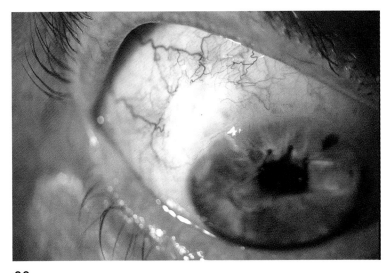

99. This is the appearance of an eye following glaucoma drainage surgery.

a. What is the type of bleb?
b. What are the conventional drainage procedures in current use?
c. What are the causes of a postoperative shallow anterior chamber?
d. What are the main late complications of drainage procedures?

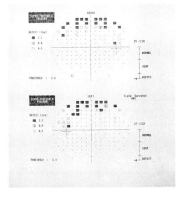

100. This is a picture of an automated visual field analysis of a 57-year-old diabetic myope, who has a family history of primary open-angle glaucoma. On examination, her intraocular pressures were 26 mmHg in each eye and the optic cup: disc ratio was 0.7 in each eye with thinning of the neuroretinal rims inferiorly.

a. How can you explain the visual field loss (dark squares)?
b. What is a Bjerrum scotoma?

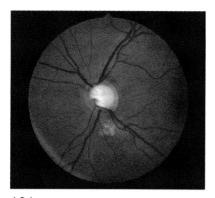

101. This 49 year-old-lady with a negative family history for primary open-angle glaucoma, was referred to the ophthalmologist because of raised intraocular pressures of 26 mm Hg in the right eye and 24 mmHg in the left eye. The visual field was normal.

a. What is the cup : disc ratio?
b. What is the normal range for intraocular pressure in the British population?
c. What is the diagnosis and management?

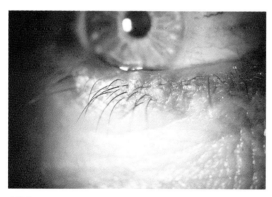

102. This 30-year-old man has had mildly sore eyes for several years.

a. What is the diagnosis?
b. What other signs may be present?
c. What is the treatment?
d. Are there any systemic associations?

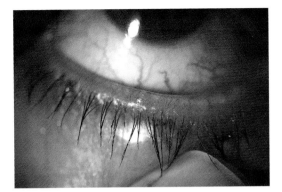

103. This 40-year-old female complains of a burning sensation in her eyes which is worse first thing in the morning.

a. What is the diagnosis?
b. How do you classify this condition?
c. What is the treatment?
d. Are there any systemic associations?

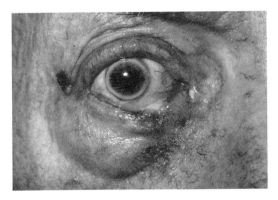

104. This is a 67-year-old man with a large squamous cell carcinoma of his lower eyelid.

a. What is the lymphatic drainage of the eyelids?
b. Which skin lesions predispose to squamous cell carcinoma?
c. In order of frequency which malignant tumours may affect the eyelids?

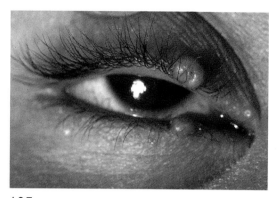

105. This 15-year-old girl has had a sore eye for 6 weeks.

a. What is the diagnosis?
b. What is the causative agent?
c. What is the cause of her symptoms?
d. What is the treatment?
e. What are potential long-term complications of untreated cases?

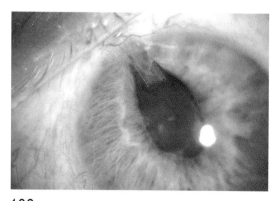

106. This is the appearance of an eye following the insertion of an artificial filtering shunt.

a. What are the main indications for this procedure?
b. What devices are in current use?
c. What are the main complications of this procedure?

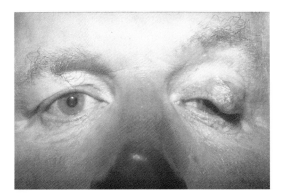

107. This patient has had a sebaceous gland carcinoma on the left upper eyelid for 8 months.

a. From which eyelid and periocular structures may the tumour originate?
b. What are the main clinical types?
c. What is meant by pagetoid spread?
d. What is her prognosis for life?

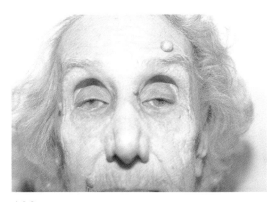

108. This 85-year-old lady developed bilateral ptosis several years ago.

a. What are the clinical features?
b. How would you classify her type of ptosis?
c. What are the other types of ptosis and give one example of each?
d. What are the main operations to correct ptosis?

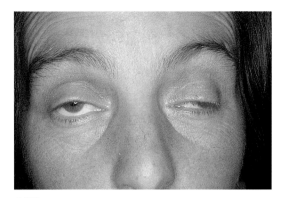

109. This 40-year-old female with myasthenia presented with bilateral ptosis and intermittent vertical diplopia.

a. What are the main clinical types of myasthenia?
b. What investigations are appropriate in suspected cases?
c. What other systemic disease may give rise to ptosis?

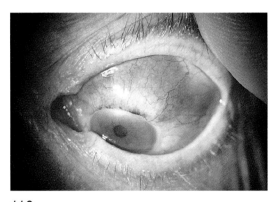

110. This 64-year-old female developed this gradually enlarging conjunctival tumour over 4 months.

a. What are the clinical signs?
b. What is the differential diagnosis?
c. How can the diagnosis be established?

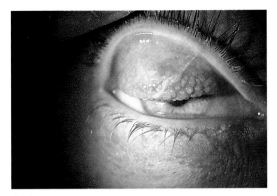

111. This is the eye of a 12-year-old boy who developed severe ocular itching and photophobia 8 months ago.

a. What are the sings?
b. What is the probable diagnosis?
c. Are there any systemic associations?
d. What corneal complications may occur?

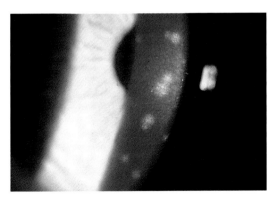

112. This is the cornea of a 34-year-old patient with adenoviral keratoconjunctivitis.

a. Which viruses are most frequently responsible for the infection?
b. What is the incidence of keratitis?
c. What is the sequence of the corneal changes?
d. What is the role of topical steroid therapy?

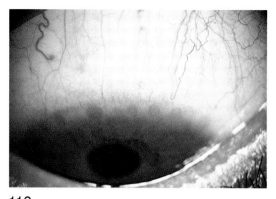

113. This is the limbus of a 45-year-old patient with inactive trachoma.

a. What are these lesions called?
b. What is their pathogenesis?
c. What is the WHO grading of trachoma?
d. What other ocular infections are caused by chlamydia?

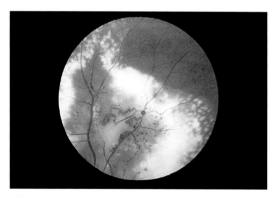

114. This is the fundus of a 9-year-old boy with Coats' disease.

a. What are the signs?
b. What is the mode of inheritance?
c. How does the condition present?
d. What are the other types of retinal telangiectasis?

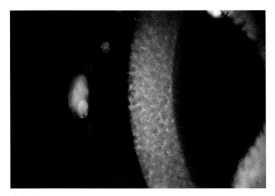

115. This is the cornea of a 20-year-old man who developed recurrent corneal erosions at the age of 5 years.

a. What is the diagnosis?
b. What is the mode of inheritance?
c. What is the underlying enzyme deficiency?
d. What is the long-term visual prognosis?

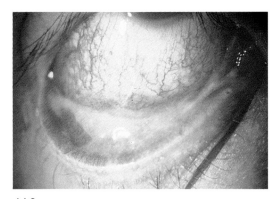

116. This white lesion formed in the lower fornix during an attack of conjunctivitis. It was peeled off easily leaving the epithelium intact.

a. What is the lesion?
b. What are the possible causes?
c. What is the differential diagnosis?

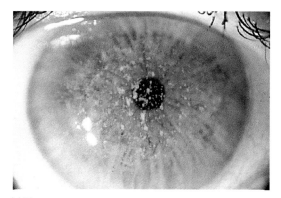

117. This is the cornea of a 19-year-old female who developed recurrent corneal erosions at the age of 7 years.

a. What is the diagnosis?
b. What is the mode of inheritance?
c. What are possible systemic associations?
d. What are the staining characteristics?
e. What is her likely visual acuity when she is 40 years old?

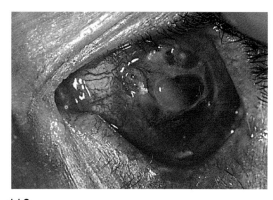

118. This is an eye with advanced Mooren's ulcer.

a. What are the two main types of this condition?
b. What are the treatment options?
c. Which systemic disorders may be associated with peripheral corneal thinning and ulceration?

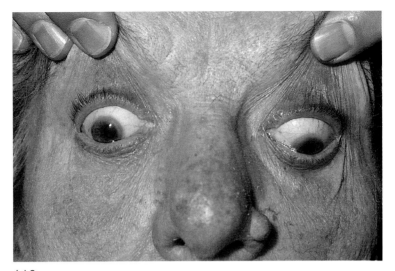

119. This 63-year-old diabetic female developed sudden onset double vision and a right incomplete ptosis. The photograph was taken when she was looking down.

a. What are the signs?
b. What is the probable diagnosis?
c. What are the most common causes?
d. What are uncommon causes?

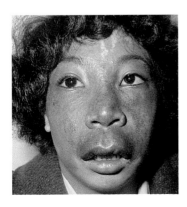

120. This 20-year-old female has had bilateral glaucoma surgery.

a. What is the systemic diagnosis?
b. What is the mode of inheritance?
c. What is the possible mechanism of her glaucoma?
d. What other ocular lesions may be present?

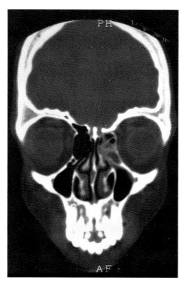

121. This is the CT scan of a woman who struck her left eye against the corner of a table.

a. Through which plane has the scan been taken?
b. What is the abnormality?
c. How do these patients usually present?
d. What is the management?

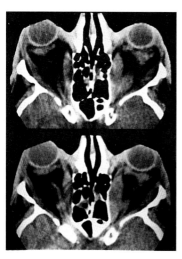

122. This is a CT scan of a 58-year-old woman who complains of diplopia and reduction of vision in her left eye.

a. Through which plane have the scans been taken?
b. What is the abnormality?
c. Does this explain her symptoms?
d. What is the most likely diagnosis?

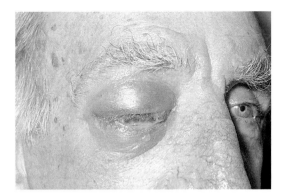

123. This 68-year-old diabetic presented with a painful swelling of the left eye 2 days after an insect bite on his left upper eyelid. The lids could not be sufficiently separated to allow adequate ocular examination.

a. What is the diagnosis?
b. What is a possible fatal complication?
c. What is the management of this case?

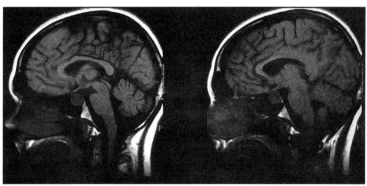

124. This is a MRI scan of a 52-year-old man who had bitemporal visual field loss.

a. Through which plane have the scans been taken?
b. What do the terms T1 and T2 weighted MRI scan mean?
c. Which is this?
d. What is the finding?

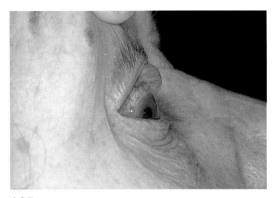

125. This woman was found to have an intraocular pressure of 26 mmHg in this eye 3 weeks after trabeculectomy.

a. What is the diagnosis?
b. Why is the intraocular pressure raised?
c. What are the treatment options?

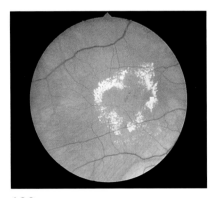

126. This is the fundus of a 48-year-old non-insulin-dependent diabetic.

a. What sign is shown?
b. Does this necessarily warrant treatment?
c. What are the 5 features of background diabetic retinopathy?

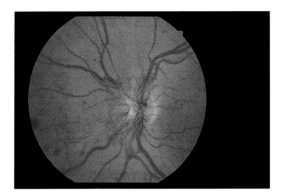

127. This is the optic disc of a 34-year-old insulin-dependent diabetic.

a. What are the signs?
b. What is the HLA association with insulin-dependent diabetes mellitus?
c. What clinical features increase the 2-year risk of developing severe visual loss (worse than 6/60)?
d. What is the treatment?

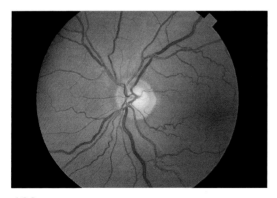

128. This is the fundus of a 60-year-old hypertensive female.

a. What are the findings?
b. What is arteriosclerosis?
c. What are the grades of hypertensive retinopathy?

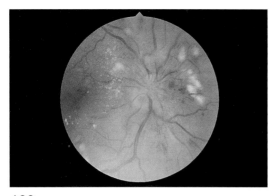

129. This is the fundus of a 40-year-old hypertensive man.

a. What is the grade of hypertensive retinopathy?
b. What is the grade of hypertension?
c. What other fundus changes may occur in hypertensives?
d. What other ocular complications may occur?

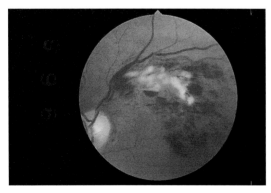

130. This patient presented with a sudden unilateral blurring in vision.

a. What is the diagnosis?
b. What complications may arise?
c. What is the pathogenesis?

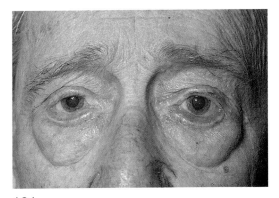

131. This 78-year-old patient complains of watering and sore eyes.

a. What is the diagnosis?
b. Why should the patient's eyes be watering?
c. How do you classify this condition?

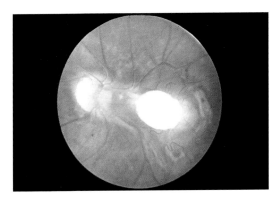

132. This 11-year-old boy presented with decreased vision in the affected eye.

a. What is the diagnosis?
b. How may this condition present systemically?
c. In which other ways may this condition affect the eye?

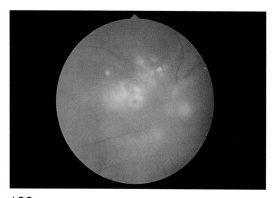

133. This is a 28-year-old woman who has been feeling run down recently and presented with blurred vision and photophobia.

a. What are the signs?
b. What is the likely cause of her symptoms?
c. Is the fact that she has been feeling run down significant?

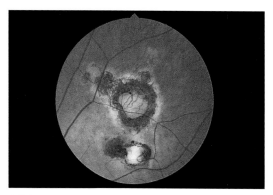

134. This 43-year-old man was referred by his optometrist, who found this asymptomatic fundus lesion.

a. What is the probable diagnosis?
b. Which animal is the definitive host for the organism responsible?
c. What are the features of the disease caused by infection with this organism in utero?

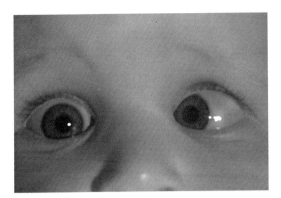

135. This 6-month-old girl was noted to have an esotropia at the age of 2 months.

a. What are the main clinical features of infantile esotropia?
b. What is the initial management?
c. What potential problems may arise subsequently?

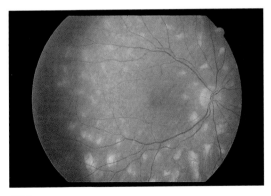

136. This is the fundus of a healthy 45-year-old woman who has noticed increasing vitreous floaters for the last 9 months. She is a carrier of HLA-A29.

a. What is the likely diagnosis?
b. What is the underlying metabolic defect?
c. What vision-threatening complications may arise?
d. What is the treatment?

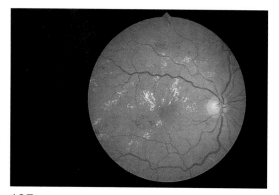

137. This is a fundus showing severe background diabetic retinopathy in a 65-year-old non-insulin-dependent diabetic. Slitlamp biomicroscopy with a +78D lens shows that he has clinically significant macular oedema.

a. How is retinal oedema recognized clinically?
b. What is the definition of macular oedema?
c. What is the definition of clinically significant macular oedema?

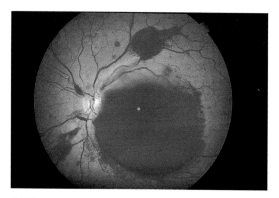

138. This is the fundus of a 35-year-old diabetic with proliferative retinopathy who recently noted a sudden and severe loss of his central vision.

a. What are the signs?
b. Is strict diabetic control beneficial in patients with diabetic retinopathy?
c. What factors may adversely affect diabetic retinopathy?

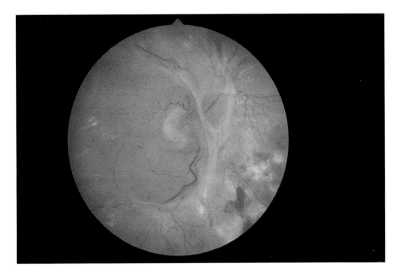

139. This is the fundus of a 35-year-old insulin-dependent diabetic who is being considered for vitrectomy.

a. What are the signs?
b. What are the main aims of vitrectomy in proliferative diabetic retinopathy?
c. What are the main indications for vitrectomy in patients with proliferative diabetic retinopathy?

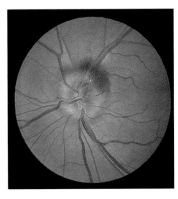

140. This is the fundus of an asymptomatic 49-year-old man.

a. What is the diagnosis?
b. Is the lesion likely to increase in size?
c. Is this patient's life threatened?
d. Is this patient's sight threatened?
e. What is the treatment?

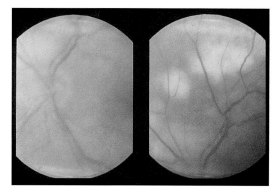

141. This is the fundus of a 68-year-old female who developed vitreous floaters in this eye 6 months ago. She was diagnosed as having intermediate uveitis but did not respond to steroid therapy. She now complains of very severe headaches.

a. What is the likely diagnosis?
b. What may be the cause of her headaches?
c. What is the risk of involvement of the second eye?
d. What is the treatment?

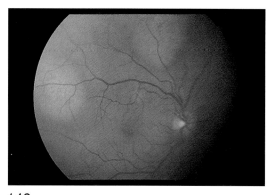

142. This fundus shows two choridal metastases.

a. What is the most common primary tumour site in females?
b. What is the most common primary site in males?
c. Which primary tumour frequently metastasizes to the orbit but very rarely to the choroid?
d. What is the management?
e. Apart from melanoma and metastases, what other tumours arise from the choroid?

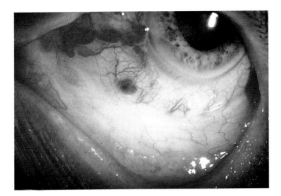

143. This shows extraocular extension of a ciliary body melanoma.

a. In what other ways may ciliary body melanomas present?
b. What diagnostic tests may be useful?
c. What other tumours may arise from the ciliary body?

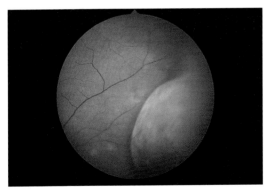

144. This is a large choroidal melanoma.

a. What are the treatment options?
b. What are adverse prognostic factors?

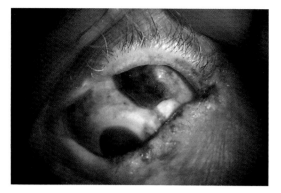

145. This is a large malignant melanoma of the conjunctiva.

a. What are the 3 main clinical and pathological types?
b. What is the overall mortality rate?
c. What are adverse prognostic factors?
d. What are the treatment options?

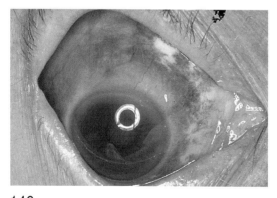

146. This is an example of congenital ocular melanocytosis.

a. At what level is the hyperpigmentation?
b. What is the risk of malignant transformation?
c. What other lesions may be present?

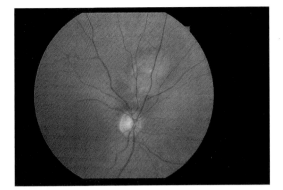

147. This shows a choroidal lesion that may be a small melanoma.

a. What clinical features would be suggestive of malignancy?
b. What special investigations may be appropriate in this case?

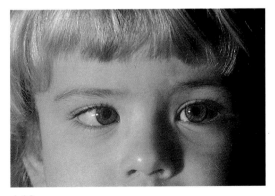

148. This girl has a manifest right convergent squint.

a. What is the classification of childhood esotropia?
b. What are the main types of amblyopia?
c. By what methods can amblyopia be treated?

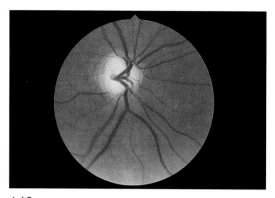

149. This 42-year-old diabetic myope was found to have raised intraocular pressure by his optometrist.

a. What is the cup : disc ratio?
b. How many nerve fibres are present in a normal optic disc?
c. What conditions may predispose a patient to developing primary open-angle glaucoma?
d. Does this patient have primary open-angle glaucoma?

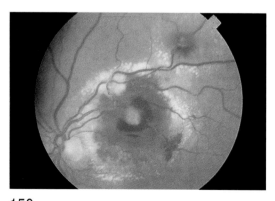

150. This is the fundus of a 73-year-old hypertensive female with gradual visual impairment.

a. What is the diagnosis?
b. What are the causes of visual impairment in this condition?
c. What is the treatment?

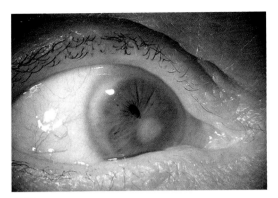

151. This is the eye of a 6-year-old child with nystagmus. The condition is bilateral and has been present since birth.

a. What is the diagnosis?
b. What is the mode of inheritance?
c. What are other associated ocular anomalies?
d. What systemic defects may be present?

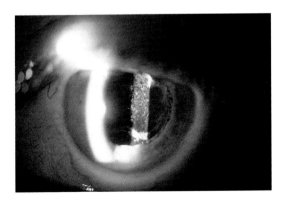

152. This patient developed opacification of the posterior capsule 9 months following uneventful extracapsular cataract extraction.

a. What are the main types of postoperative capsular opacification?
b. What are the indications for Nd:YAG laser capsulotomy?
c. What is the safest time to perform capsulotomy?
d. What are the potential complications of laser capsulotomy?

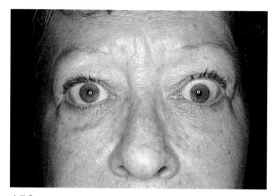

153. This is a 56-year-old female with thyroid opthalmopathy.

a. What are the lid signs in thyroid eye disease?
b. Which surgical procedures can be used to correct severe lid retraction?
c. What are non-thyroid causes of lid retraction?

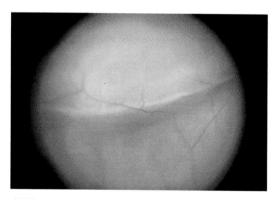

154. This is a ring choroidal detachment in a patient with posterior scleritis.

a. What are the other clinical signs of posterior scleritis?
b. What are the main conditions that should be considered in the differential diagnosis of posterior scleritis?
c. What are the main clinical differences between a retinal and a choroidal detachment?

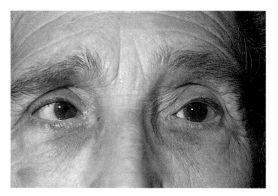

155. This 62-year-old man has failure of abduction of the left eye due to a sixth nerve palsy.

a. What are the clinical features of Foville's syndrome?
b. What are the clinical features of Millard–Gubler syndrome?
c. What are important causes of a basilar sixth nerve palsy?

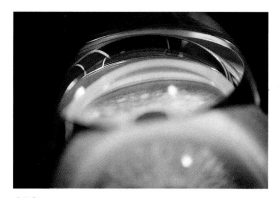

156. This is a gonioscopic view of a wide open angle with a pigmented trabecular meshwork.

a. What are the causes of trabecular hyperpigmentation?
b. What are the main types of gonioscopes?
c. What is grade 2, according to the Shaffer grading?

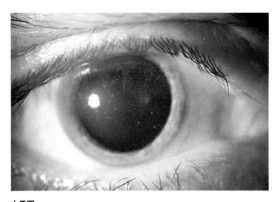

157. This is the eye of a 34-year-old man who was found to have a visual acuity of 6/18 by his optometrist due to cataract. The fellow eye was normal.

a. What are the clinical features?
b. What is the probable diagnosis?
c. What other anterior segment signs may be present?
d. What is the management of this patient's eye condition?

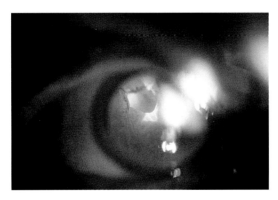

158. This is an eye with a retinal detachment due to a large 'U'-shaped tear.

a. What are the complications of drainage of subretinal fluid?
b. What are the main causes of early failure of a scleral buckling procedure?
c. What are the main causes of subsequent re-detachment following initially successful surgery?

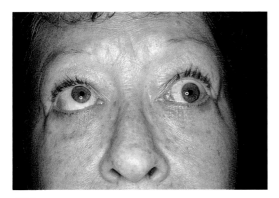

159. This patient has diplopia associated with thyroid ophthalmopathy.

a. What is the pathogenesis of diplopia in thyroid ophthalmopathy?
b. In order of frequency what ocular motility defects may be present?
c. What are the indications for orbital decompression?
d. What are the main types of orbital decompression?

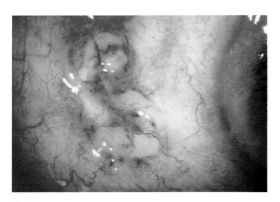

160. This is the eye of a patient with necrotizing scleritis with inflammation.

a. What is the treatment?
b. What are possible underlying systemic associations?
c. What is the treatment of non-necrotizing anterior scleritis?

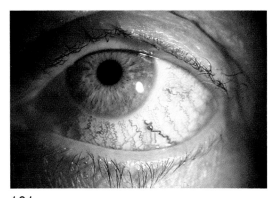

161. This 72-year-old hypertensive female developed sudden headache and a red eye.

a. What is the probable diagnosis?
b. What may cause this condition?
c. What other signs may she develop?
d. What are the causes of 'dynamic' proptosis?

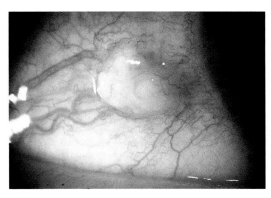

162. This is the eye of a 19-year-old girl who developed discomfort and photophobia 2 days ago.

a. What is the likely diagnosis?
b. What is the pathogenesis?
c. What complications may occur?
d. What is the treatment?
e. What is the differential diagnosis?

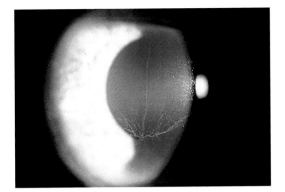

163. This is the cornea of an asymptomatic 40-year-old female.

a. What is the diagnosis?
b. From what systemic disease may she be suffering?
c. What associated retinal changes may be present?

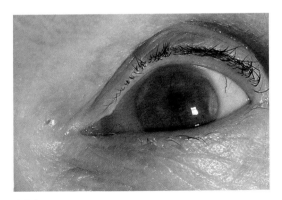

164. This is the cornea of an 8-year-old girl with chronic arthritis.

a. What is the diagnosis?
b. What is the likely cause in this patient?
c. What are other causes of this condition?
d. What are the treatment options, if required?

165. This is a skin lesion of an 18-year-old girl with bilateral iris nodules.

a. What is the skin lesion?
b. What is the probable systemic diagnosis?
c. How is the systemic condition classified?
d. What is the differential diagnosis of congenital iris nodules?

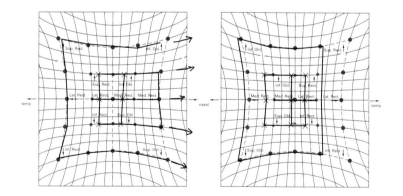

166. This is a Hess chart of a hypertensive diabetic who presented with sudden-onset painless diplopia.

a. What principle is used in a Hess chart to pinpoint a muscle paresis?
b. On which side is the paretic muscle and why?
c. Is this test accurate if the patient has abnormal retinal correspondence?

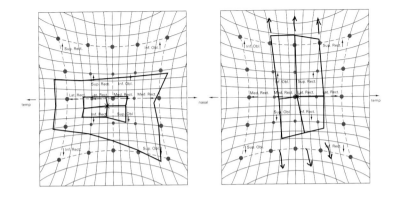

167. This is a Hess chart of a 21-year-old man who received a blow to the left eye and subsequently developed diplopia.

a. What are the signs?
b. How can you differentiate between an innervational and a mechanical defect on a Hess Chart?
c. What is the likely diagnosis?

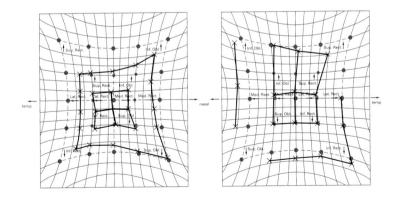

168. This is a Hess chart of a 49-year-old lady who complains of diplopia.

a. What are the signs?
b. Is this likely to be a mechanical or innervational defect?
c. What is the most likely diagnosis?

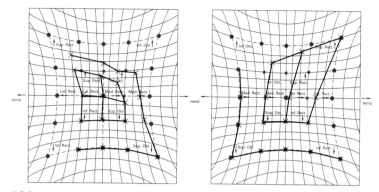

169. This is a Hess chart of a 10-year-old boy.

a. What pattern of horizontal deviation is this?
b. Is this a left inferior oblique palsy?
c. What is the likely diagnosis?
d. What is the aetiology of this condition?

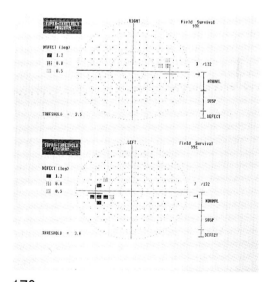

170. This is an automated visual field analysis.

a. What does 'suprathreshold program' mean?
b. What is the visual field defect?
c. What are the causes of such a defect?

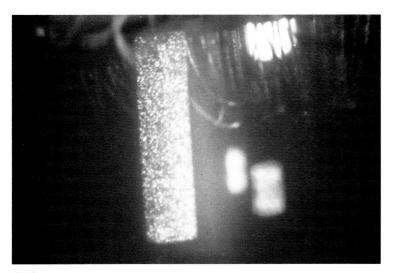

171.

a. Describe the signs.
b. What is the possible aetiology?

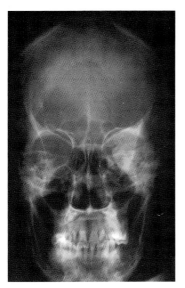

172. This is a skull X-ray of a 42-year-old woman who presented with a 4-month history of gradually worsening proptosis and visual acuity on the affected side.

a. What is the finding?
b. What are the causes of this finding?

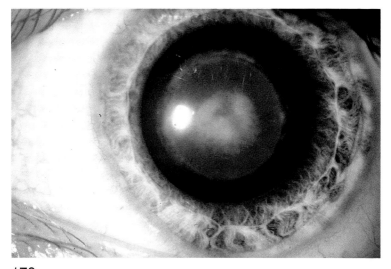

173. This child has bilateral congenital cataracts.

a. How might the child present to the ophthalmologist?
b. What is the aetiology?

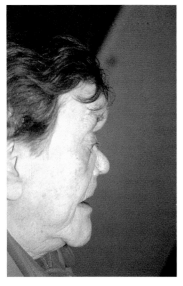

174. This 68-year-old lady has bilateral nerve deafness.

a. Describe her facies.
b. What congenital disorder may she have?
c. What ocular manifestations may she have?

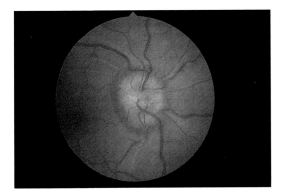

175. This 44-year-old lady presented with a 2-year history of headaches and worsening vision together with 'noises in her head'. MR scanning was completely normal.

a. Describe the signs.
b. What is the diagnosis?
c. What other symptoms may patients with this condition have?
d. What additional investigation is required?

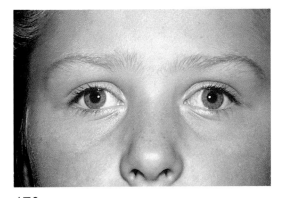

176. This child is fixing with her right eye on an object in the distance.

a. What is the diagnosis?
b. What are the cover tests?

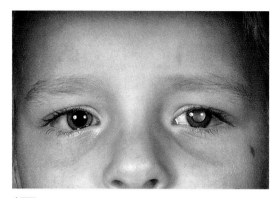

177. This child was noted to have an absent red reflex.

a. What is the diagnosis until excluded?
b. What else could it be?

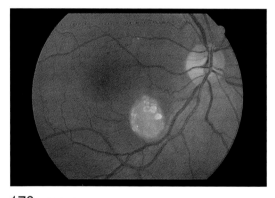

178. This is the fundus of a 10-year-old boy with epilepsy.

a. What is the lesion shown?
b. What is the probable cause of his epilepsy?
c. What is the mode of inheritance?
d. What skin lesions may be present?

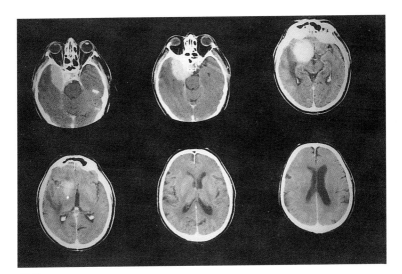

179. This patient presented with a progressive decrease in vision of his right eye. He had a mild right relative afferent pupillary defect and decreased colour vision. His right disc was pale, but not cupped.

a. What does the CT scan show and what is the diagnosis?
b. Is the fact that there was no proptosis surprising?
c. From which cells does this tumour arise?
d. What feature if seen histologically is suggestive of this tumour?

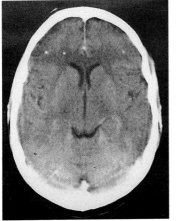

180. This young man presented with unilateral blurred vision due to a focal retinochoroiditis, followed by a confusional state.

a. Describe the signs.
b. What is the differential diagnosis?
c. What underlying conditions need to be excluded?

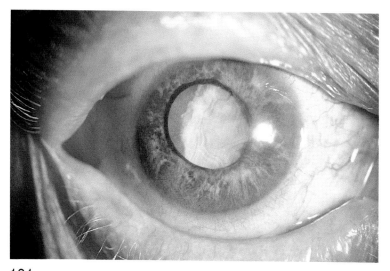

181. This 75-year-old man has hand movements vision in the eye shown. He noticed gradual deterioration of vision over 4–5 years.

a. How do you classify cataracts?
b. What type of cataract is this?
c. What are the methods of cataract extraction?

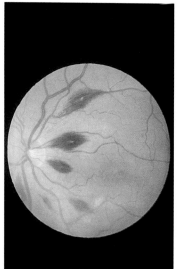

182. This is the fundus of a 35-year-old man who has been unwell for over a month.

a. What is the sign?
b. What could be the underlying systemic disease?
c. What are the hyperviscosity syndromes?

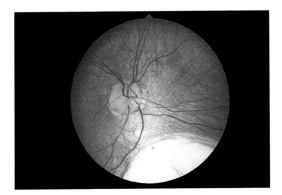

183. This is a retinochoroidal coloboma.

a. How does it form?
b. Is this a typical example?
c. What percentage are bilateral?

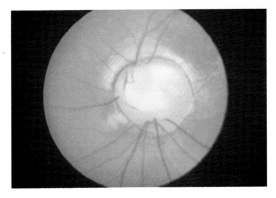

184. This patient has poor vision and an altitudinal field defect.

a. What is the diagnosis?
b. What are the ocular associations?
c. What are the systemic associations?

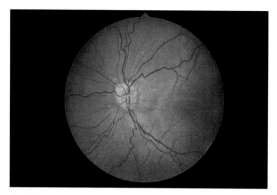

185. **This is the fundus of a patient referred by an optometrist who suspected papilloedema.**

a. What features suggest this is not papilloedema?
b. What is the likely diagnosis if the optic disc showed autofluorescence?
c. What is the differential diagnosis of swollen discs?

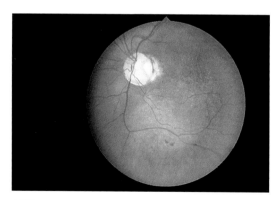

186. **This is the fundus of a 38-year-old man who developed blurred vision and metamorphopsia one year ago which spontaneously resolved after 5 months. His present visual acuity is 6/12.**

a. What is the fundus diagnosis?
b. What was the likely cause of his visual symptoms?
c. What is the pathogenesis of this complication?
d. What is the risk to the other eye?

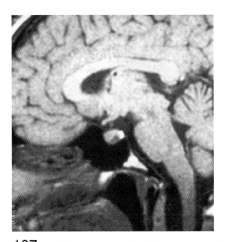

187. This MR scan is of a 28-year-old male with a central scotoma in one eye and loss of the superotemporal field in the other eye.

a. Why is there an area highlighted within the pituitary?
b. The type of visual disturbance pattern described has a name. What is it?
c. What are the main differences between MR and CT scans?

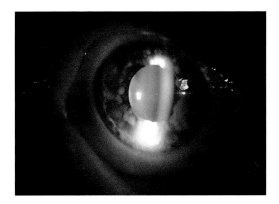

188. This is the eye of a 4-year-old whose father had one eye enucleated as a child.

a. Describe the appearance of the iris.
b. What is the likely diagnosis?
c. Can you explain the genetics of this condition?

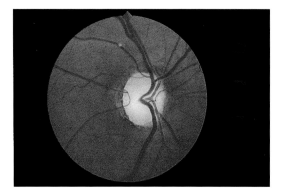

189. **This 72-year-old patient has counting fingers vision in both eyes and the appearance of both of his optic discs is identical.**

a. What is the sign?
b. What is the aetiology of this when it is bilateral and acquired?
c. What is the aetiology when it is unilateral?

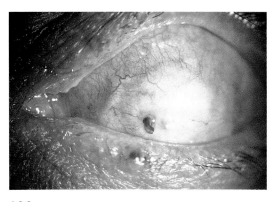

190. **This patient was allegedly attacked with ammonia 3 months ago.**

a. What is the mechanism of damage?
b. What is the initial treatment for alkali injuries to the eyes?

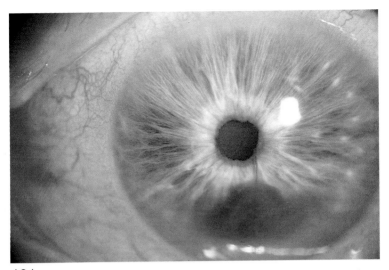

191. This patient presented with loss of vision in the affected eye and no history of trauma.

a. What is the diagnosis?
b. What is the aetiology?

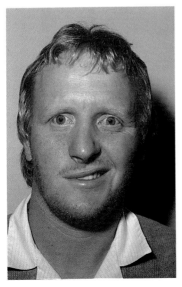

192. This man developed sensorineural deafness on the same side as this upper motor neurone facial nerve palsy.

a. Which clinical reflex would you wish to perform?
b. What is the reason?
c. If this reflex is absent which investigations are appropriate?

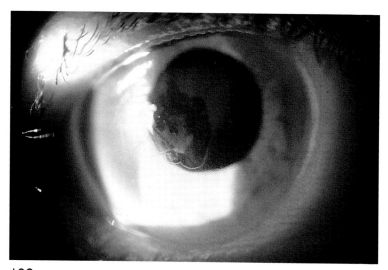

193. This is the eye of a 75-year-old lady with an irritable eye and slight photophobia.

a. What is the diagnosis?
b. What is the pathogenesis?
c. What is the most common cause encountered in clinical practice?
d. What are other causes?
e. What is the management?

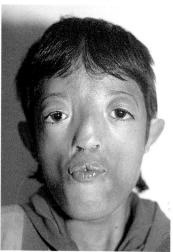

194. This child has the rare Robert's syndrome comprising bilateral proptosis (secondary to shallow orbits), midline craniofacial anomalies and hypomelia.

a. What are the more common causes of shallow orbits?
b. What are the other causes of bilateral proptosis in a child?

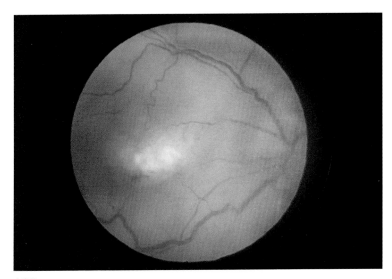

195. This is the fundus of a 34-year-old man who complains of floaters with blurring of vision for 3 weeks.

a. Why does the lesion appear hazy?
b. What are the possible causes?
c. What is the dye test?
d. What is its significance if positive?

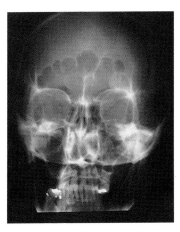

196. This is the skull X-ray of a 62-year-old female who had a mastectomy 2 years ago.

a. Could the lesion above the left orbit be a metastasis?
b. What is the differential diagnosis?
c. Which primary tumours may metastasize to the bony orbit?

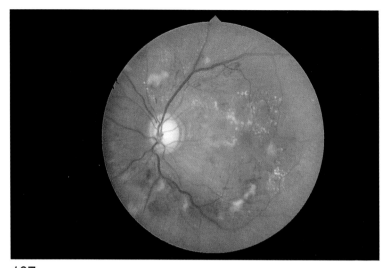

197. This **57-year-old insulin-dependent diabetic noticed blurred vision in this eye.**

a. What are the main types of diabetic retinopathy?
b. What type is shown?
c. What is your management of this case?

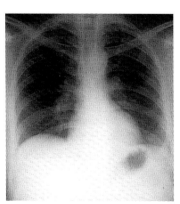

198. This is the chest X-ray of a **33-year-old man with a positive Kveim test.**

a. What are the signs?
b. What is the probable systemic diagnosis?
c. What eyelid lesions may occur in this condition?
d. What anterior segment complication may he subsequently develop?

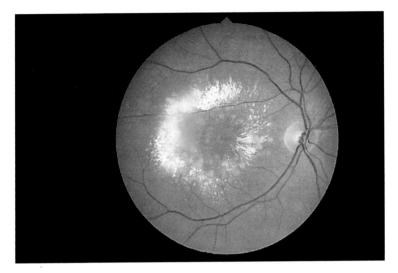

199. **This fundus shows extensive deposition of hard exudates.**

a. What is the basic pathogenesis of hard exudate formation?
b. How would you classify the main causes?

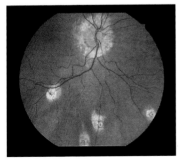

200. **This is the fundus of a 35-year-old patient with metamorphopsia who has lost his central vision due to the presumed ocular histoplasmosis syndrome.**

a. What is the probable cause of his visual loss?
b. What could be his tissue typing?
c. What are the vitreous changes in this condition?
d. What are other causes of multifocal inflammatory lesions affecting the fundus?

Answers

1.
  a. Choroideremia. The mode of inheritance is X-linked recessive so that affected males cannot pass the gene to their sons but all daughters are carriers.
  b. Choroideremia is not associated with any known biochemical abnormality.
  c. His mother will be a carrier and will have mild fundus changes in the form of patchy peripheral retinal atrophy and mottling of the retinal pigment epithelium.

2.
  a. Gyrate atrophy of the retina and choroid.
  b. Patients with gyrate atrophy have an inborn error of the mitochondrial matrix enzyme ornithine-delta-aminotransferase. This leads to increased levels of ornithine in the plasma, urine, cerebrospinal fluid and aqueous. Treatment with pyridoxine (vitamin B_6) and a diet low in proteins and arginine may be beneficial.
  c. The mode of inheritance is autosomal recessive.
  d. Patients with gyrate atrophy may also have:
    • myopia
    • vitreous degeneration
    • cystoid macular oedema
    • complicated cataract.

3.
  a. The macula shows a 'bicycle wheel-like' appearance pathognomonic of congenital retinoschisis. With time visual acuity continues to decline and non-specific atrophic macular changes ensue.
  b. The inheritance is X-linked recessive.
  c. Between 50–70% of patients with macular schisis also have peripheral retinoschisis in which the inner leaf is extremely thin and consists only of the internal limiting membrane and the retinal nerve fibre layer. Complications of peripheral retinoschisis are:
    • large defects in the inner layer—very common
    • virtreous haemorrhage—uncommon
    • retinal detachment—uncommon.
  d. Nil.

4.
  a. The signs are:
    • complete lack of fundus pigment
    • absence of foveal landmarks
    • optic disc hypoplasia.
  b. Tyrosinase-negative (complete) oculocutaneous albinism.

   c. Other abnormalities include:
- a diaphenous blue iris that transilluminates completely
- myopic or hypermetropic refractive errors
- strabismus
- anomalous retinogeniculate projections so that many of the temporal hemiretinal fibres decussate in the chiasm with the nasal hemiretinal fibres.

   d. Two potentially lethal forms of albinism are:
- Chédiak–Higashi syndrome characterized by susceptibility to infections
- Hermansky–Pudlak syndrome with a predisposition to bruising and bleeding.

5.
a. Best's vitelliform macular dystrophy.
b. Inheritance is autosomal dominant with variable penetrance and expressivity.
c. The five stages of Best's disease are:
Stage 1—previtelliform (normal fundus but abnormal EOG)
Stage 2—vitelliform (egg-yolk stage) as shown in this case
Stage 3—pseudohypopyon (part of lesion becomes absorbed)
Stage 4—vitelliruptive (scrambled-egg)
Stage 5—end stage is characterized by one of the following:
- hypertrophic macular scar
- atrophic macular scar
- vascularized fibrous macular scar.

d. Visual acuity is usually no worse than 6/60.

6.
a. Choroidal naevus.
b. Most choroidal naevi are hypofluorescent due to blockage of background choroidal fluorescence.
c. Over 90% of choroidal naevi are located posterior to the equator.
d. Very rare complications of choroidal naevi are:
- secondary choroidal neovascularization
- malignant transformation.

7.
a. Myelinated nerve fibres.
b. The condition is not hereditary.
c. The condition is bilateral in about 20% of cases.
d. Males are more frequently affected.
e. Vision may be affected as follows:
- by macular involvement with reduction of visual acuity
- peripheral myelination will cause corresponding scotomas which may be relative or absolute.

8.
a. Krukenberg spindle.
b. Pigmentary glaucoma.
c. Pigmentary glaucoma is not hereditary.

     d. Other anterior segment features include:
- slit-like iris transillumination defects
- an excessively deep anterior chamber with a posterior bowing of the midperipheral iris
- circumferential hyperpigmentation of the posterior trabecular meshwork
- pigment granules within iris furrows and on both surfaces of the lens.

9.
a. Congenital ectropion uveae.
b. The patient should have regular measurement of intraocular pressure because a significant percentage of cases develop glaucoma between early childhood and puberty due to an associated angle anomaly.
c. Neurofibromatosis type 1.

10.
a. Asteroid hyalosis.
b. Most eyes with asteroid hyalosis have normal or near normal visual acuity.
c. Most patients do not have any underlying systemic disease although a small percentage may have diabetes.
d. Cholesterolosis bulbi (synchysis scintillans) differs from asteroid hyalosis because:
- It is usually unilateral whilst asteroid hyalosis is bilateral in 25% of cases.
- It usually follows a vitreous haemorrhage.
- The particles are more mobile within the vitreous.

11.
a. Tilted discs.
b. Tilted discs are not inherited.
c. Eyes with tilted discs frequently have associated inferonasal ectasia of the fundus which gives rise to upper temporal visual field defects. However, unlike the field defects due to chiasmal compression, they do not obey the vertical midline.
d. The headaches are incidental.

12.
a. Pediculosis. The picture shows nits (eggs laid by the female) firmly attached to the lashes.
b. The eyelashes should be smothered with liquid paraffin and the nits physically peeled off with cotton wool buds. This should be done every day for a week.
c. Pediculosis humanis has three main varieties:
- capitis—infesting the head
- corporis—infesting the body and clothes
- pubis—infesting the genital and other hairy parts of the body.

13.
a. No; since these are the only lesions and there is no dermatomal distribution to the vesicular eruption.
b. Primary herpes simplex infection.
c. The ophthalmic ointment contains a much lower concentration of acyclovir than the cream. The cream should therefore be applied directly to the lesions but care should be taken to avoid the eyes.

14.
a. Traumatic right superior oblique palsy.
b. The compensatory head posture would be:
   - head tilt to the left
   - face turn to the left
   - chin depression.
c. When appropriate, surgical correction will depend on whether hypertropia or torsion is the main deviation.
   - For hypertropia:
     - (i) weakening of the ipsilateral inferior oblique, or
     - (ii) weakening of the contralateral inferior rectus.
   - For torsion (excyclotropia):
     - (i) Harada–Ito procedure, or
     - (ii) plication of the paretic muscle.

15.
a. Severe rubeosis iridis.
b. Ischaemic central retinal vein occlusion.
c. Neovascular glaucoma caused by secondary synechial angle-closure by fibrovascular tissue in the angle. This typically develops about three months following central retinal vein occlusion (100-day glaucoma).
d. Other causes of rubeosis iridis are:
   - Proliferative retinopathies
     - (i) diabetic—the risk is increased by cataract and vitreous surgery
     - (ii) sickle cell disease.
   - Carotid artery disease including carotid-cavernous fistula.
   - Chronic intraocular inflammation.

16.
a. Left Brown's superior oblique tendon sheath syndrome.
b. Ten percent of cases are bilateral.
c. Most congenital cases do not require treatment. Indications for surgery include the presence of a hypotropia in the primary position and an anomalous head posture. The most frequently used procedure is superior oblique tenotomy with or without ipsilateral inferior oblique recession.
d. Similar motility defects may be due to:
   - acquired Brown's syndrome due to trauma or tenosynovitis of the superior-oblique-trochlear apparatus

- inferior oblique palsy
- entrapment of the inferior oblique muscle in a blow-out fracture of the orbital floor.

17.
a. Anterior ischaemic optic neuropathy. This is a segmental or generalized infarction within the prelaminar or laminar portion of the optic nerve caused by occlusion of the posterior ciliary arteries.
b. The three main causes of anterior ischaemic optic neuropathy are as follows:
   - Giant cell arteritis is a common cause in the elderly.
   - The non-arteritic type typically occurs in hypertensive individuals between the ages of 45–65 who have absent or small optic cups.
   - Auto-immune optic neuropathy occurs in younger patients with systemic lupus erythematosus or some other collagen vascular disease.
c. In this elderly patient it is important to exclude the possibility of giant cell arteritis by performing:

erythrocyte sed. rate

   - ESR—a normal value does not necessarily exclude giant cell arteritis.
   - Test for C-reactive protein which is invariably raised in giant cell arteritis.
   - Temporal artery biopsy to obtain histological confirmation.

18.
a. Buphthalmos (large eyes) and left exotropia.
b. Autosomal recessive with incomplete penetrance.
c. Gonioscopy shows absence of the angle recess with either a flat or a concave insertion of the iris into the surface of the trabecular meshwork.
d. Treatment of most cases is by goniotomy with a success rate of about 85%.
e. The main causes of visual impairment are:
   - optic nerve damage
   - anisometropic amblyopia
   - corneal scarring
   - cataract
   - lens subluxation.

19.
a. Duane's syndrome type-1 characterized by limitation of abduction but normal adduction.
b. About 20% of cases are bilateral.
c. Some children with Duane's syndrome have perceptive deafness with an associated speech disorder.

d. Most cases do not require surgery. Indications for surgery are:
   - to overcome an anomalous head posture
   - to enlarge the field of single binocular vision
   - to correct cosmetically unacceptable upshoots or down shoots.

20.
a. Central retinal vein occlusion.
b. The three main types of central retinal vein occlusion are:
   - ischaemic
   - non-ischaemic
   - in young adults.
c. Underlying factors may be systemic and ocular.
   - Systemic underlying factors include:
     (i)   old age
     (ii) hypertension
     (iii) blood dyscrasias associated with hyperviscosity.
   - Ocular factors include:
     (i)   raised intraocular pressure
     (ii) congenital anomaly of the central retinal vein
     (iii) periphlebitis as in Behçet's disease and sarcoidosis.

21.
a. The main atypical types of retinitis pigmentosa are:
   - sector—involving one quadrant or one half of each fundus
   - with exudative vasculopathy—bilateral telangiectatic vascular anomalies, serous retinal detachment and lipid deposition in the retinal periphery
   - pericentric
   - retinitis punctata albescens.
b. The three main macular lesions are:
   - atrophic maculopathy
   - cellophane maculopathy
   - cystoid macular oedema which may respond to acetazolamide.
c. Associated ocular lesions include:
   - optic disc drusen
   - open-angle glaucoma
   - posterior subcapsular cataracts
   - keratoconus
   - myopia
   - intermediate uveitis.

22.
a. Stargardt's fundus flavimaculatus.
b. Inheritance is usually autosomal recessive.
c. The four main patterns are:

- maculopathy without flecks
- maculopathy with perifoveal flecks
- maculopathy with diffuse flecks (as shown here)
- diffuse flecks without maculopathy.

d. There are no associated ocular lesions.

23.
a. Lacquer cracks are large breaks in Bruch's membrane.
b. The main types of maculopathy are:
   - myopic degeneration involving the macula
   - neovascular maculopathy associated with lacquer cracks
   - macular haemorrhage unassociated with lacquer cracks
   - macular hole.
c. Other ocular complications are:
   - vitreous degeneration
   - rhegmatogenous retinal detachment due to either macular or peripheral retinal holes
   - posterior staphylomas
   - increased prevalence of primary open-angle glaucoma and steroid responsiveness
   - posterior subcapsular cataract and early onset nuclear sclerosis.
d. Uncommon systemic associations include:
   - Marfan's syndrome.
   - Ehlers–Danlos syndrome.
   - Stickler's syndrome.

24.
a. Occlusion of the cilioretinal artery.
b. Emboli can be seen in both the superior and inferior branches of the artery. The possible causes of retinal embolism are:
   - Carotid artery disease which may give rise to three types of emboli:
     - (i) cholesterol (Hollenhorst's plaques)
     - (ii) fibrinoplatelet
     - (iii) calcific.
   - Heart disease which may give rise to four types of emboli:
     - (i) calcific from calcified valves
     - (ii) valve vegetations in SBE (subacute bacterial endocarditis)
     - (iii) thrombus from the left atrium
     - (iv) from an atrial myxoma.
c. The ischaemic retina appears white due to cloudy swelling involving the retinal nerve fibre and ganglion cell layers. Because the fovea itself is devoid of these layers the orange reflex from the intact choroidal vessels beneath the fovea stands out in contrast to the surrounding opaque retina.

25.
a. Congenital hypertrophy of the retinal pigment epithelium.
b. Hereditary polyposis coli which may be associated with one of the following:
  - Gardner's syndrome—osteomas and soft tissue abnormalities
  - Turcot's syndrome—neuroepithelial brain tumours.
c. Autosomal dominant.
d. The patient should have a colonoscopy and, if found to have polyposis, prophylactic colectomy should be performed because of the very high risk of adenocarcinoma of the colon.

26.
a. Fundus albipunctatus.
b. Inheritance is autosomal recessive.
c. The long-term visual prognosis is excellent because the macula remains unaffected.
d. The main conditions that should be considered in the differential diagnosis of a flecked retina are:
  - familial dominant drusen—most common by far
  - fundus flavimaculatus
  - retinitis punctata albescens
  - flecked retina of Kandori.

27.
a. Malignant melanoma of the iris.
b. The differential diagnosis of iris melanoma includes:
  - Other tumours
    - (i) large iris naevus
    - (ii) leiomyoma
    - (iii) juvenile xanthogranuloma
    - (iv) metastasis.
  - Iris cysts
    - (i) primary
    - (ii) secondary to intraocular surgery.
  - Large inflammatory granuloma.
c. The prognosis is excellent because the predominant cell type is usually spindle-B.
d. The treatment options are:
  - broad iridectomy for localized tumours such as this
  - iridocyclectomy or iridotrabeculectomy for larger tumours involving the angle
  - enucleation, rarely required for diffusely growing tumours.

28.
a. Ectopia lentis is a displacement of the lens from its normal anatomical position.
b. • Luxation is a complete displacement of the lens from the pupillary space.

- Subluxation is a partial displacement in which a part of the lens still remains within the pupillary space.
  c. Syndromes associated with ectopia lentis are:
    - Marfan's syndrome—subluxation is typically up
    - Weill–Marchesani syndrome—lens is small and spherical (microspherophakia) and subluxation is down
    - Stickler's syndrome—10% have lens subluxation
    - Ehlers–Danlos syndrome—subluxation is uncommon.
  d. Metabolic disorders associated with ectopia lentis are:
    - homocystinuria—subluxation is down
    - hyperlysinaemia
    - sulphite oxidase deficiency.

29.
  a. Lisch nodules.
  b. The nodules are melanocytic naevi composed of proliferations of spindle cells of neural crest origin.
  c. Neurofibromatosis type-1.
  d. The most likely cause of the proptosis and optic atrophy is an optic nerve glioma which develops in about 15% of patients.
  e. Other ophthalmic lesions in neurofibromatosis-1 are:
    - Eyelid neurofibromata
    - Orbital lesions
        (i) neural orbital tumours (neurilemmoma, plexiform neurofibroma, meningioma)
        (ii) spheno-orbital encephalocele.
    - Intraocular lesions
        (i) prominent corneal nerves
        (ii) congenital glaucoma
        (iii) congenital ectropion uveae
        (iv) choroidal hamartomas
        (v) optociliary shunt vessels in eyes with optic nerve tumours.

30.
  a. Iris coloboma.
  b. The condition is usually not hereditary.
  c. The pathogenesis is failure of fusion of the apex of the embryonic fissure.
  d. Possible associated ocular anomalies are:
    - colobomas of the ciliary body, lens, choroid and optic nerve
    - microcornea.
  e. Potential systemic associations are:
    - Goldenhar's syndrome
    - Treacher Collins syndrome
    - Cat's eye syndrome
    - Rubenstein–Taybi syndrome

- CHARGE syndrome (Colobomatous microphthalmia, Heart anomaly, Atresia choanal, Retarded growth, Genital and Ear anomalies).

31.
a. A non-filtering flat vascularized bleb.
b. Potential causes of failure of filtration are:
  - subconjunctival fibrosis
  - accelerated wound healing associated with intraocular inflammation
  - inadequate sclerostomy
  - blockage of the sclerostomy by blood, Descemet's membrane, uveal tissue, or vitreous.
c. The success rate of filtration may be enhanced by:
  - corticosteroids which suppress postoperative inflammation
  - antimetabolites such as 5-fluorouracil and mitomycin which prevent fibroblast proliferation
  - excision of Tenon's capsule.

32.
a. Commotio retinae (Berlin's oedema) involving the posterior pole.
b. The natural course of commotio retinae is either:
  - complete resolution—most common
  - development of microcystoid degeneration of the outer retinal layers
  - development of retinoschisis from breakdown of the septa in the microcysts.
c. Other posterior segment complications of blunt trauma are:
  - avulsion of the vitreous base and tearing of the non-pigmented epithelium of the pars plana
  - retinal dialysis
  - peripheral retinal holes
  - macular hole
  - choroidal rupture.

33.
a. Clinically the severity of ptosis is graded by measuring the marginal reflex distance, bearing in mind that the upper eyelid covers between 1.5–2 mm of the cornea.
  - mild ptosis = 2 mm or less
  - moderate ptosis = 3 mm (as in this patient)
  - severe ptosis = 4 mm or more.
b. Levator function is assessed by measuring the upper lid excursion. It is graded as follows:
  - good = 12 mm or more
  - fair = 6–11 mm (as in this patient)
  - poor = 5 mm or less.
c. The ideal time to operate is between the ages of 3 and 4.

d. Treatment is by levator resection assuming there is simple congenital ptosis not associated with the jaw-winking phenomenon.

34.
a. The fundus shows cicatricial retinopathy of prematurity characterized by dragging of the blood vessels and macular heterotopia.
b. Threshold disease includes:
  • stage 3 retinopathy of prematurity
  • involvement of zone 1 or 2
  • evidence of 'plus' disease
  • involving 5 or more continuous clock hours or 8 cumulative clock hours.
c. Screening schedule:
  • Initial, between 4–7 weeks postnatally.
  • Follow-up
    (i) if normal fundi, every 2 weeks until 36 weeks
    (ii) if zone 1 or 2 disease present, weekly.

35.
a. Partial aniridia.
b. The four phenotypes of aniridia are:
  • with normal vision
  • associated with poor vision due to foveal hypoplasia (as in this case)
  • associated with Wilm's tumour of the kidney
  • associated with mental retardation.
c. The inheritance pattern may be:
  • autosomal dominant associated with the first two phenotypes
  • autosomal recessive associated with mental retardation
  • sporadic, associated with Wilm's tumour with deletion of the short arm of chromosome 11.
d. Other possible ocular defects in aniridia.
  • Glaucoma develops from the second decade of life in 50% of cases.
  • Cornea—opacity, microcornea, sclerocornea, keratolenticular adhesions
  • Lens—cataract, subluxation, congenital absence, persistent pupillary membranes
  • Posterior segment—foveal hypoplasia, choroidal coloboma, hypoplastic discs.

36.
a. Crouzon's syndrome is a craniofacial synostosis characterized by proptosis due to shallow orbits.
b. The two main causes of poor vision in Crouzon's syndrome are:

- optic atrophy caused by bony compression of the optic nerves in the optic canal
- exposure keratopathy.

c. Other ocular defects include:
  - hypertelorism and exotropia
  - luxation of the globe
  - nystagmus, either primary or secondary to poor vision.

d. No; mental retardation is uncommon.

37.
a. Left Horner's syndrome—ptosis and miosis.
b. The main congenital causes of heterochromia are:
  - idiopathic
  - Horner's syndrome
  - Waardenburg's syndrome
  - Sturge–Weber syndrome.
c. The main acquired causes of heterochromia are:
  - Fuchs' heterochromic cysclitis
  - diffuse iris tumours (naevi, melanoma, juvenile xanthogranuloma)
  - pigment dispersion syndrome
  - siderosis
  - severe rubeosis iridis
  - progressive facial hemiatrophy.

38.
a. Amaurosis fugax which is a retinal transient ischaemic attack.
b. Arcus lipoides (often mistakenly referred to as arcus senilis in patients under the age of 60). Both conditions are caused by deposition of non crystalline cholesterol although the former is associated with type II and III hyperlipidaemias and the latter is a change associated with age.
c. Type I—hyperchylomicronaemia
   Type IIa—familial hypercholesterolaemia
   Type IIb—mixed hyperlipidaemia
   Type III—broad beta disease
   Type IV—familial hypertriglyceridaemia
   Type V—hyperchylomicronaemia and familial hypertriglyceridaemia.
d. • Directly: xanthelasma (II & III); lipaemia retinalis (I, III, IV & V)
   • Indirectly: accelerated atherosclerosis leads to atheromatous carotid artery disease, which predisposes to retinal artery occlusion, homonymous hemianopia due to a cerebrovascular accident and ocular ischaemia.

39.
a. Lattice degeneration.
b. Rare systemic associations are:

- Stickler's syndrome
- Marfan's syndrome
- Ehlers–Danlos syndrome.

c. The main indications for prophylactic treatment are:
- retinal detachment in the fellow eye
- extensive lattice in a highly myopic eye
- strong family history of retinal detachment
- the three systemic conditions mentioned above.

d. Macular pucker (preretinal gliosis).

40.
a. Herpes zoster ophthalmicus.
b. Treatment is as follows:
- oral acyclovir, 800 mg 5 times daily for 7 days
- an antibiotic-steroid preparation (e.g. Neo-Cortef ointment or Terra-Cortil spray) applied directly to the skin lesions.

c. The main acute ocular lesions that may impair vision are:
- iritis which may be associated with secondary glaucoma
- punctate epithelial keratitis
- microdendritic ulceration
- nummular keratitis
- optic neuritis (rare).

d. Apart from optic neuritis, uncommon neurological complications are:
- cranial nerve palsies
- encephalitis
- contralateral hemiplegia.

41.
a. Traumatic hyphaema.
b. Other anterior segment injuries of blunt trauma are:
- rupture of the iris sphincter
- scleral rupture
- laceration of the anterior face of the ciliary body (angle-recession), which may be associated with subsequent secondary glaucoma
- lens subluxation or dislocation.

c. The main current vision-threatening complications are:
- secondary glaucoma
- blood staining of the cornea, which may occur if the intraocular pressure is over 25 mm Hg for more than 6 days.

d. Management is as follows:
- admission to hospital for strict bed rest and regular monitoring of intraocular pressure
- treatment of secondary glaucoma, if present
- topical steroids; the role of mydriatics is controversial

- surgical evacuation of the blood clot if corneal blood staining threatens.

42.
a. Type 1 lattice corneal dystrophy.
b. Autosomal dominant.
c. The material is amyloid.
d. The material stains with congo red.
e. This patient has type 1 lattice dystrophy which is not associated systemic disease. However, patients with type 2 lattice dystrophy, which does not present with recurrent corneal erosions, have systemic amyloidosis.

43.
a. Pseudoexfoliative glaucoma (glaucoma capsulare).
b. About 20% of initially normal fellow eyes develop glaucoma within 10 years.
c. Pseudoexfoliative material is thought to be derived from the iris.
d. Sampaolesi's line is a scalloped band of pigment running onto or anterior to Schwalbe's line which is virtually pathognomonic of pseudoexfoliation.
e. The zonules may rupture during cataract surgery.

44.
a. Squamous cell papilloma.
b. Removal is by simple surgical excision with cauterization to the base to prevent recurrence.
c. The salient histological features are:
    - finger-like projections of vascularized connective tissue
    - acanthotic epidermis with elongated rete ridges
    - areas of hyperkeratosis and focal parakeratosis within the epidermis.
d. Other benign eyelid tumours are:
    - seborrhoeic keratosis—basal cell papilloma
    - molluscum contagiosum
    - strawberry naevus
    - port wine stain
    - keratoacanthoma
    - pigmented naevi
        - –intradermal
        - –junctional
        - –compound
    - inverted follicular keratosis.

45.
a. A post-traumatic subconjunctival haemorrhage such as this suggests the possibility of a fracture involving the anterior cranial fossa.
b. The Battle sign is localized bruising over the mastoid process which occurs in basal skull fractures.
c. A right afferent pupillary conduction defect is probably

present because the CT scan shows a bony fragment
impinging the right optic nerve.

46.
a. Angioid streaks.
b. Causes of visual impairment in eyes with angioid streaks are:
   - maculopathy secondary to choroidal neovascularization
   - traumatic choroidal rupture causing a subfoveal
     haemorrhage
   - foveal involvement by an angioid streak.
c. Pseudoxanthoma elasticum, although it is possible that the
   haemorrhage is incidental.
d. About 50% of patients have no systemic disease. Systemic
   associations in order of importance include:
   - Pseudoxanthoma elasticum (Gronblad–Strandberg
     syndrome).
   - Paget's disease.
   - Haematological disorders
     - (i) homozygous sickle cell disease
     - (ii) thalassaemia
     - (iii) thrombocytopenic purpura.
   - Miscellaneous
     - (i) acromegaly
     - (ii) senile elastosis
     - (iii) facial angiomatosis
     - (iv) lead poisoning.

47.
a. Incontinentia pigmenti (Bloch–Sulzberger syndrome)—a
   mesodermal and ectodermal dysplasia affecting girls.
b. X-linked dominant.
c. Systemic manifestations are:
   - vesiculobullous dermatitis that resolves spontaneously
     leaving irregular patches or whorls of hyperpigmentation
     (shown here)
   - variable malformations of teeth, hair, nails, bones and
     central nervous system.
d. Leukocoria is due to fibrovascular proliferation leading to
   cicatricial retinal detachment.

48.
a. Blow-out fracture of the orbital floor.
b. Associated clinical signs include:
   - periocular ecchymosis, oedema and occasionally
     emphysema
   - enophthalmos
   - infraorbital nerve anaesthesia
   - diplopia which typically occurs in both downgaze and
     upgaze
   - ocular damage—uncommon.

c. Initial management involves:
- administration of systemic antibiotics to prevent spread of infection from the maxillary sinus to the orbit
- baseline Hess test to assess muscle restriction
- baseline exophthalmometry to assess degree of enophthalmos.

d. The main indications for surgery are large fractures involving half or more of the orbital floor, particularly if associated with severe enophthalmos and persistent significant diplopia in the primary position.

49.
a. Limbal dermoid.
b. Goldenhar's (oculoauricular vertebral) syndrome:
- deafness
- multiple vertebral anomalies
- depressed lateral orbital rims, maxillary and mandibular hypoplasia
- wide mouth
- microtia and preauricular skin tags.

c. Other ocular lesions in Goldenhar's syndrome are:
- upper eyelid and iris colobomas
- microcornea, microphthalmos and anophthalmos
- tilted disc and optic nerve hypoplasia
- macular hypoplasia
- strabismus.

50.
a. Central retinal artery occlusion.
b. Immediate management is:
- Lie patient flat.
- Give intravenous acetazolamide 500 mg.
- Apply firm ocular massage intermittently for at least 15 minutes.
- Other measures include:
  - (i) inhalation of a mixture of 5% carbon dioxide and 95% oxygen
  - (ii) anterior chamber paracentesis.

c. Despite immediate treatment the visual prognosis in the majority of cases is extremely poor.

d. Other vascular causes are:
- Retinal vein occlusion
- Anterior ischaemic optic neuropathy
- Vitreous haemorrhage
- Premacular or macular haemorrhage.

51.
a. Entropion of the lower eyelid.
b. Classification of entropion:

- involutional—due to age-related atrophy
- acute spastic—secondary to irritation of the cornea
- cicatricial—due to scarring of the conjunctiva or eyelid
- congenital.

c. Depending on the cause, procedures to correct entropion include:
  - simple taping of the eyelid to the cheek
  - use of histoacryl
  - cautery
  - transverse lid everting suture
  - Weis procedure
  - Fox procedure
  - strengthening of lower lid retractors
  - tarsal fracture—for cicatricial entropion.

52.
a. Blepharophimosis syndrome.
b. The main signs are:
  - congenital ptosis
  - epicanthus inversus
  - telecanthus—a lateral soft tissue displacement of the medial canthi
  - mild ectropion of the lower lids.
c. Where appropriate, initial treatment involves correction of the epicanthus and telecanthus followed later by correction of ptosis with a frontalis suspension procedure.

53.
a. Bell's phenomenon.
b. It is absent in 10% of normal eyes.
c. Exposure keratopathy.
d. Prevention of exposure keratopathy.
  - Temporary measures:
    - (i) frequent instillation of lubricating agents
    - (ii) taping of eyelids at night
    - (iii) temporary tarsorrhaphy
    - (iv) botulinum toxin.
  - Permanent measures:
    - (i) medial canthoplasty
    - (ii) graded levator recession
    - (iii) prosthetic devices.

54.
a. The meanings of the histological terms are as follows:
  - Hyperkeratosis is increased keratinization within the skin.
  - Acanthosis is an increase in the prickle cell layer due to increase in mitotic activity of the basal cells.
  - Papillomatosis is a pattern of growth where sheets of cells cover a surface.

b. Seborrhoeic keratosis—also referred to as basal cell papilloma, seborrhoeic wart and senile verruca.

c. Because it is not a premalignant condition removal is purely on cosmetic grounds.

d. Four premalignant eyelid lesions are:
  • actinic keratosis
  • Bowen's disease
  • lentigo maligna
  • cutaneous horn which may be associated with an underlying actinic keratosis or squamous cell carcinoma.

55.
a. The most likely diagnosis (taking into account the appearance of the lesion and its slow growth rate) is basal cell carcinoma.

b. The risk of metastasis in a basal cell carcinoma is extremely small.

c. A basal cell carcinoma occurring in a young person demands careful follow-up to ensure it is not the first sign of the Gorlin–Goltz syndrome (basal cell naevus syndrome). This is an autosomal dominant disorder in which there are multiple basal cell carcinomas associated with cysts of the jaw, skeletal anomalies, neurological abnormalities and endocrine disorders.

56.
a. Keratoacanthoma.

b. Indirectly; because keratoacanthoma occurs with increased frequency in immunosuppressed individuals.

c. Spontaneous resolution is common but may take up to a year.

d. Surgical excision is advised because occasionally keratoacanthoma shows histological evidence of invasive squamous cell carcinoma at deeper levels of section.

57.
a. Xanthelasma, which is a xanthoma occurring on the eyelid.

b. Nil.

c. About one-third of patients with xanthelasma have either primary or secondary hyperlipidaemia.

d. Xanthomata may also occur on the skin of buttocks (eruptive type), on extensor surfaces (tuberous type), in palmar creases and on tendons.

58.
a. Central tarsorraphy (suturing together of the lids).

b. The main indications are severe exposure keratopathy or intractable corneal ulcer (usually neuropathic).

c. Botulinum toxin A may be injected under electromyographic control into the levator palpebrae superioris.

59.
a. Endophthalmitis due to bleb infection.
b. The thin-walled cystic bleb with a positive Siedel test is particularly vulnerable because it drains transconjunctivally.
c. Management:
  - admit to hospital
  - take aqueous and vitreous cultures
  - intraocular injection of vancomycin and amikacin
  - topical cefuroxime and fortified vancomycin or gentamicin
  - systemic ceftazidime and/or ciprofloxacin
  - topical steroids.

60.
a. Capillary haemangioma.
b. Removal is only indicated if there is a threat of amblyopia, either by the tumour obstructing the visual axis or by inducing severe astigmatism.
c. The Kasabach–Merritt syndrome is the association of haemangiomas with thrombocytopaenic purpura. The syndrome usually occurs in infants and the onset of purpura is accompanied by rapid enlargement of the tumour. Its pathogenesis is believed to be linked to sequestration of platelets within the tumour and associated visceral angiomas.

61.
a. Acute anterior uveitis.
b. In anterior uveitis there is an intense mononuclear cell infiltration of the iris, ciliary body and ciliary muscle. Exposure to bright light induces ciliary muscle spasm.
c. Provided the patient is appropriately treated the visual prognosis is very good. The main vision threatening complication is the formation of posterior synechiae which may lead to secondary pupil block glaucoma. In a small proportion of patients the uveitis becomes chronic.

62.
a. An inflammatory arthropathy affecting mainly young males, 70% of whom are HLA B27 positive. The classic triad is of urethritis, conjunctivitis and arthritis. Patients may also get balanitis or buccal ulceration. Other features are plantar fasciitis, keratoderma blenorrhagia and nail dystrophy. About 20% of patients develop recurrent attacks of acute anterior uveitis.
b. Because of the very severe anterior chamber reaction the patient should be given an anterior sub-Tenon's injection of steroid. The pupil should be dilated with intensive mydriatics. Topical steroid drops should also be prescribed at very frequent intervals.
c. Calcification within the Achilles' tendon near its insertion, the so-called calcaneal spur.

63.
a. Mutton fat keratic precipitates.
b. A fusiform distribution of keratic precipitates in the lower half of the cornea.
c. Granulomatous.
d. Koeppe and Busacca nodules.
e. Causes of granulomatous uveitis:
   - sarcoidosis
   - tuberculosis
   - sympathetic ophthalmitis
   - Vogt–Koyanagi–Harada syndrome
   - toxoplasmosis
   - syphilis
   - lens-induced uveitis
   - late-onset postoperative endophthalmitis due to Proprionibacterium acnes.

64.
a. Rieger's anomaly.
b. Autosomal dominant.
c. About 50% of patients develop glaucoma, usually during early childhood.
d. Some patients with Rieger's anomaly have Rieger's syndrome which is associated with the following systemic lesions:
   - dental anomalies—small teeth (microdontia) and a decrease in number of teeth (hypodontia)
   - facial malformations—hypoplasia of maxilla, telecanthus, flat nasal bridge and hypertelorism.

65.
a. Filamentary keratitis.
b. Corneal filaments are composed of mucus threads attached at one end to abnormal corneal epithelium.
c. Causes of filamentary keratitis are:
   - keratoconjunctivitis sicca
   - superior limbic keratoconjunctivitis
   - herpes zoster ophthalmicus
   - essential blepharospasm
   - midbrain strokes.

66.
a. Bacterial, chlamydial and viral.
b. Treatment of bacterial conjunctivitis:
   - Norfloxacin (Noroxin) has a broad spectrum with low toxicity and a prolonged effect so that four times daily use is sufficient.
   - Ofloxacin (Exocin) has similar properties.
   - Fucidic acid (Fucithalmic) is useful for staphylococcal infection.
   - Other drugs include: gentamicin, framycetin, tobramycin and chloramphenicol.

     c. Systemic associations:
- hay fever
- atopic dermatitis
- Reiter's disease
- ocular cicatricial pemphigoid
- Stevens–Johnson syndrome
- epidermolysis bullosa
- thyroid dysfunction—superior limbic keratoconjunctivitis.

67.
a. There is a white superior corneal infiltrate which is separated from the limbus by a clear zone.
b. Marginal keratitis.
c. Probably; because in patients with staph. blepharitis the keratitis is thought to be caused by a hypersensitivity reaction to Staphylococcal exotoxins.
d. Treatment is with a short course of a weak steroid such as fluorometholone or clobetasone provided the possibility of herpes simplex infection has been excluded.

68.
a. Optic atrophy.
b. The main hereditary optic atrophies are:
- Leber's hereditary optic neuropathy which typically affects young males.
- Autosomal dominant optic atrophy (Kjer type)—onset 4–8 years.
- Autosomal recessive optic atrophies:
    - (i) simple—onset 2–3 years
    - (ii) complicated (Behr's syndrome)—onset 1–9 years and associated with neurological abnormalities
    - (iii) associated with other defects such as diabetes mellitus, diabetes insipidus, deafness and ataxia.
c. The Foster–Kennedy syndrome consists of unilateral optic atrophy and contralateral papilloedema. It is classically caused by a subfrontal tumour which causes ipsilateral optic atrophy by direct compression and contralateral papilloedema due to raised intracranial pressure.

69.
a. Cytomegalovirus retinitis.
b. The cytomegalovirus is an opportunistic infection which only affects immunocompromised individuals, especially those with AIDS.
c. The treatment of cytomegalovirus retinitis is with either intravenous gancyclovir or foscarnet. The former can also be administered intravitreally by injections or slow-release devices.

    d. Other fundus lesions in immunocompromised individuals are:
- pneumocystis carinii choroidopathy
- cryptococcus choroiditis
- severe toxoplasma retinochoroiditis
- varicella-zoster retinitis
- large cell intraocular lymphoma.

70.
a. Optic nerve hypoplasia.
b. The condition is not inherited.
c. His ataxia may be caused by one of the following:
- Neurological malformations—basal encephalocele, hypoplasia of the cerebellar vermis, cystic dilatation of the fourth ventricle, posterior fossa cysts and anterior visual pathway space-occupying lesions.
- De Morsier's syndrome (septo-optic-dysplasia)—short stature and midline developmental anomalies (absence of septum pellucidum, agenesis of corpus callosum, and dysplasia of the anterior third ventricle).

d. Other ocular anomalies in eyes with optic nerve hypoplasia are:
- microphthalmos
- absence of the foveal reflex
- aniridia.

71.
a. Steroid induced geographic (amoeboid) herpes simplex ulceration. In this patient the inadvertent use of topical steroids has prevented the host response from combating the viral infection so that it has become rampant with the formation of a large ulcer.
b. The steroids should be stopped and the patient treated with topical acyclovir ointment five times a day until the ulcer has healed.
c. The continued use of topical steroids in this eye could have led to severe complications in the form of stromal necrotic keratitis with subsequent vascularization, scarring and even perforation.

72.
a. Treatment of acute glaucoma is as follows:
- Prophylactic pilocarpine 1% q.i.d. to the fellow eye.
- Administration of systemic pressure-lowering therapy such as intravenous acetazolamide or an oral (isosorbide, glycerol) or intravenous (mannitol) hyperosmotic agent.
- Topical therapy with:
  - (i) pilocarpine 2%
  - (ii) β-blocker
  - (iii) steroids.

- Peripheral laser iridotomy once the cornea has cleared.
- Prophylactic laser iridotomy to the fellow eye.
  b. The classification of primary angle-closure glaucoma is as follows:
  - latent
  - intermittent (subacute)
  - acute—congestive and post-congestive
  - chronic
  - absolute.
  c. The three main mechanisms of chronic angle-closure glaucoma are:
  - gradual and progressive (creeping) synechial angle-closure
  - following several intermittent attacks
  - a combination of primary open-angle glaucoma with narrow angles.

73.
a. Pterygium.
b. There is no racial predisposition but pterygia typically occur in people living in hot climates.
c. Indications for removal are:
  - cosmetic
  - recurrent inflammation and irritation
  - progressive growth towards the visual axis.
d. The methods of preventing recurrences are:
  - operative use of mitomycin C
  - postoperative β-irradiation
  - treatment of early recurrences with the argon laser.
e. A true pterygium should be differentiated from a pseudopterygium which is caused by adhesion of a fold of conjunctiva to a peripheral corneal ulcer.

74.
a. Superior limbic keratoconjunctivitis of Theodore.
b. Thyroid function tests would be appropriate because between 20 and 50% of patients have associated thyroid dysfunction.
c. Treatment options are:
  - Correction of thyroid dysfunction, if present.
  - Topical therapy with—
    (i) adrenaline 1% for symptomatic relief
    (ii) acetylcysteine 5% to reduce filamentary keratitis
    (iii) tear substitutes for associated dry eyes.
  - Soft bandage contact lenses.
  - Thermocauterization of the superior bulbar conjunctiva.
  - Superior limbal conjunctival resection.

75.
a. Corneal abrasion.
b. Because fluorescein has been used. The dye remains extracellular and because it stains the tear film it shows up epithelial corneal defects as bright green when examined under cobalt blue light.
c. This patient may subsequently develop the recurrent erosion syndrome due to improper hemidesmosome formation between the basement membrane and epithelium. Diabetics are at increased risk of developing this condition.

76.
a. He may be right because topical adrenaline derivatives may result in adrenochrome deposits in the conjunctiva.
b. No.
c. Yes, because adrenaline is a phenol that is oxidized to adrenochrome by naturally occurring oxidases and then finally to melanin.

77.
a. The differential diagnosis is:
  • herpes simplex stromal keratitis
  • bacterial keratitis
  • fungal keratitis
  • acanthamoeba keratitis.
b. The most likely diagnosis is stromal necrotic herpes simplex keratitis because:
  • Corneal sensation is reduced in herpetic infection.
  • There is no apparent predisposing factor to bacterial keratitis.
  • There is no past history of trauma with organic matter which may precede a fungal infection.
  • Acanthamoeba keratitis is unlikely because it typically occurs in contact lens wearers.
c. Treatment consists of:
  • healing of any associated epithelial defect
  • judicious use of topical steroids with antiviral and antibiotic cover.

78.
a. Herpes simplex dendritic ulcer.
b. The drugs currently available to treat active herpetic epithelial disease are:
  • acycloguanosine (Acyclovir, Zovirax) 3% ointment 5 times a day
  • trifluorothymidine 1% drops 2-hourly
  • atenine arabinose 3% ointment or 0.1% drops
  • idoxuridine 0.5% ointment or 0.1% drops
  • bromovinyldeoxyuridine 1% ointment and 0.1% drops.
c. Causes of pseudodendritic ulceration are:
  • herpes zoster keratitis

- healing corneal abrasion
- toxic keratopathy from excessive drop administration
- contact lens wear.

79.
a. Cotton-wool spot.
b. Cotton-wool spot formation is caused by occlusion of precapillary arterioles in the retinal nerve fibre layer. The ischaemia interrupts axoplasmic flow and results in the build-up of transported material within the nerve axon which is responsible for the white appearance of these lesions.
c. The main clinical causes of cotton-wool spots are:
   - retinal vein occlusion
   - preproliferative diabetic retinopathy
   - hypertensive retinopathy
   - papilloedema
   - collagen vascular disorders such as dermatomyositis, systemic lupus erythematosus and polyarteritis nodosa
   - human immunodeficiency virus retinopathy
   - haematological disorders such as anaemia, leukaemia and hyperviscosity states.

80.
a. Idiopathic (age-related) macular hole.
b. There is a 1 : 10 risk to the fellow eye.
c. There is no risk of retinal detachment.
d. Other causes of macular hole formation are:
   - blunt ocular trauma.
   - highy myopia—may give rise to retinal detachment
   - solar retinopathy may cause a very small lamellar hole or cyst.

81.
a. There is central corneal haze and thickening together with fine keratic precipitates (KP) on the endothelial surface.
b. The above findings, together with corneal anaesthesia, point to the likely diagnosis of herpetic disciform keratitis (a hypersensitivity reaction to viral antigen).
c. This is a ring around a disciform keratitis that forms as a result of immune complex deposition due to antigen diffusing radially away from the site of the keratitis and reacting with antibodies.

82.
a. Left internuclear ophthalmoplegia.
b. Other ocular motility defects in demyelination are:
   - ataxic nystagmus on abduction of the contralateral eye to the internuclear ophthalmoplegia
   - cerebellar nystagmus
   - conjugate gaze paresis
   - skew deviation
   - isolated ocular motor nerve palsies.

  c. T-2 weighted MR in patients with multiple sclerosis shows bright areas of abnormal signal in the brain stem and periventricular area. In patients with retrobulbar neuritis MR with special coils may also demonstrate a plaque within the optic nerve.

83.
a. Meibomian cyst (chalazion).
b. Predispositions are:
- acne rosacea
- seborrhoeic dermatitis.

c. The differential diagnosis:
- external hordeolum (stye)—staphylococcal infection of a lash follicle
- internal hordeolum—staphylococcal infection of a chalazion.

d. Treatment options include:
- conservative—awaiting spontaneous resolution
- incision and curettage
- injection of steroid into the lesion
- systemic antibiotics for recurrent cases associated with acne rosacea or seborrhoeic dermatitis.

84.
a. Cyst of Moll.
b. There are no known predispositions.
c. The differential diagnosis:
- cyst of Zeis—less translucent
- sebaceous cyst—has central punctum
- molluscum contagiosum—typically umbilicated.

d. Treatment:
- simple puncture with a needle
- cauterization.

85.
a. A retinal detachment is a separation of the sensory retina from the retinal pigment epithelium by subretinal fluid.
b. The main types of retinal detachment are:
- Rhegmatogenous, caused by a retinal break
  - (i) spontaneous
  - (ii) traumatic.
- Tractional, due to contracting vitreoretinal membranes
  - (i) proliferative retinopathies
  - (ii) penerating trauma.
- Exudative, due to an abnormality in the retinal pigment epithelium
  - (i) Harada's disease
  - (ii) choroidal tumours
  - (iii) toxaemia of pregnancy.

c. Long-standing rhegmatogenous retinal detachment:
- retinal tinning

- secondary intraretinal cysts
- pigment demarcation (high-water) marks
- subretinal fibrosis is occasionally present.

86.
a. This is either a subepithelial or a compound conjunctival naevus because it is slightly elevated. Junctional naevi are usually flat.
b. Virtually nil; it is common for naevi to grow and become more pigmented at puberty.
c. The two main indications for excision are:
   - cosmetic—by far the most common
   - enlargement of the lesion during adult life.
d. Other benign conjunctival tumours are:
   - papilloma
   - dermoid
   - lipodermoid
   - haemangioma.

87.
a. Symblepharon.
b. Other ocular complications of ocular cicatricial pemphigoid are:
   - keratoconjunctivitis sicca
   - eyelid deformities
     - (i) ankyloblepharon
     - (ii) entropion
     - (iii) trichiasis
     - (iv) metaplastic lashes
   - keratopathy.
c. Other causes of symblepharon are:
   - Other bullous skin diseases
     - (i) Stevens Johnson syndrome
     - (ii) epidermolysis bullosa.
   - Trauma
     - (i) chemical
     - (ii) irradiation.
   - Membraneous conjunctivitides, if inappropriately treated, may rarely give rise to symblepharon.

88.
a. Predisposing factors:
   - contact lens wear
   - trauma
   - bullous keratopathy
   - keratoconjunctivitis sicca
   - exposure keratopathy
   - neurotrophic keratopathy
   - postherapietic disease
   - chronic dacryocystitis.

b. *N. gonorrhoeae*, *C. diphtheriae*, Listeria sp., and Haemophilus sp.
c. Immediate management:
   • Take scrapings for Gram stain and culture.
   • Until results of cultures are known, treat with a combination of a topical fortified aminoglycoside (gentamicin or tobramycin) and cefuroxime or ciprofloxacin at half-hourly intervals around the clock.

89.
a. Keratoconus (conical cornea).
b. The initial form of treatment of this patient would be the fitting of contact lenses. Corneal grafting is indicated only in patients with advanced progressive disease, especially with significant corneal scarring.
c. Associated disorders may be:
   • Ocular
     (i) vernal disease
     (ii) Leber's congenital amaurosis
     (iii) retinitis pigmentosa
     (iv) aniridia
     (v) ectopia lentis.
   • Systemic
     (i) atopic dermatitis
     (ii) Down's syndrome
     (iii) Turner's syndrome
     (iv) Ehlers–Danlos syndrome
     (v) Marfan's syndrome
     (vi) osteogenesis imperfecta
     (vii) mitral valve prolapse.

90.
a. To aid in the diagnosis of possible keratoconjunctivitis sicca as it has an affinity for mucus as well as dead and devitalized cells.
b. 5 mm or less in 5 minutes.
c. 10 seconds or less.
d. Secondary Sjögren's syndrome comprises dry eyes, dry mouth and one of the following:
   • seropositive rheumatoid arthritis
   • systemic lupus erythematosus
   • systemic sclerosis
   • psoriatic arthritis
   • juvenile chronic arthritis
   • Hashimoto's thyroiditis
   • primary biliary cirrhosis.

91.
a. Metamorphopsia is a visual symptom describing disortion of shapes.

b. The angiogram shows a choroidal neovascular membrane.
c. Neovascular age-related macular degeneration.
d. Other important causes of choroidal neovascularization are:
   - idiopathic
   - high myopia
   - presumed ocular histoplasmosis syndrome
   - angioid streaks
   - optic disc drusen
   - choroidal naevus
   - choroidal rupture
   - excessive laser photocoagulation
   - Best's disease.

92.
a. Drusen (colloid bodies).
b. The five main types of drusen are:
   - hard—small
   - soft—large
   - mixed—semisolid
   - basal laminar—nodular
   - autosomal dominant
c. Histologically drusen consist of deposits of abnormal material in the inner portion of Bruch's membrane between the basement membrane of the retinal pigment epithelium and the inner collagenous layer.
d. This patient's visual prognosis is guarded because she has soft drusen which are associated with diffuse dysfunction of the retinal pigment epithelium and an increased risk of subsequently developing exudative age-related macular degeneration.

93.
a. Macular pucker (premacular gliosis).
b. Idiopathic.
c. The condition is bilateral in only 5% of cases.
d. Other causes of premacular gliosis are:
   - retinal procedures
     - retinal detachment surgery
     - laser photocoagulation
     - cryotherapy
   - retinal vascular disease
   - intraocular inflammation
   - ocular trauma.

94.
a. Bull's-eye maculopathy.
b. Long-term chloroquine medication.
c. Other causes of a bull's-eye maculopathy are:
   - cone dystrophy
   - Batten's disease

- benign concentric annular macular dystrophy
- Bardet–Biedl syndrome
- Leber's congenital amaurosis (rarely).

d. Fluorescein angiography in bull's-eye maculopathy shows a round area of hyperfluorescence around the fovea due to a window defect corresponding to the area of atrophy of the retinal pigment epithelium.

95.
a. Choroidal folds.
b. Idiopathic—frequently associated with hypermetropia.
c. Other causes of choroidal folds are:
  - orbital disease including thyroid
  - choroidal tumour
  - posterior scleritis
  - ocular hypotony.
d. The hyperfluorescence corresponding to the crests is due to a window defect associated with thinning of the retinal pigment epithelium. In contrast the retinal pigment epithelium is thicker over the troughs and therefore obscures background fluorescence.

96.
a. Morning glory anomaly.
b. The condition is not hereditary.
c. Most cases are unilateral.
d. Possible systemic associations are:
  - basal encephalocele
  - absence of the corpus callosum
  - hare lip and cleft palate.

97.
a. Juvenile chronic arthritis is an idiopathic, seronegative, inflammatory arthritis of at least 3 months duration occurring before age 16 years.
b. The main types, according to onset, are:
  - pauciarticular—four or fewer joints
  - polyarticular—five or more joints
  - systemic—fever, rash, lymphadenopathy, hepatosplenomegaly etc.
c. Risk factors for uveitis are:
  - early-onset pauciarticular
  - serum antinuclear antibodies
  - female gender
  - HLA-DW5 and HLA-DPw2.
d. Juvenile 'rheumatoid' arthritis is the counterpart of adult seropositive rheumatoid arthritis starting before the age of 16 years.

98.
a. Essential iris atrophy.
b. The condition is not hereditary.

c. Gonioscopy will show superior synechial angle closure.
d. The condition is invariably unilateral.
e. Differential diagnosis:
- iris naevus syndrome of Cogan–Reese
- Chandler's syndrome.

99.
a. A slightly avascular diffuse functioning bleb.
b. Trabeculectomy and Scheie's procedure.
c. Causes of shallow anterior chamber:
- wound leak
- excessive drainage
- ciliary shut-down
- ciliary block (malignant) glaucoma.
d. Late complications.
- bleb infection and endophthalmitis
- a slight risk of cataract formation.

100.
a. The visual field defect (scotoma) in each eye has an arcuate shape. This can be explained by loss of nerve fibres supplying the inferior retina due to glaucomatous damage consistent with thinning of the inferior retinal rim. However, such symmetrical field loss is extremely rare in primary open-angle glaucoma and other possible causes are:
- excessive skin (dermatochalasia) on upper eyelids causing obstruction of upper visual field
- very thick horn-rimmed spectacles
- retinal degenerations such as sectorial retinitis pigmentosa.
b. A paracentral scotoma that lies between 10° and 20° off fixation (Bjerrum's area).

101.
a. The vertical cup disc ratio is 0.7.
b. 10–21 mmHg.
c. Ocular hypertension (i.e. raised intraocular pressure without optic nerve damage). Regular intraocular pressure check with visual field analysis is required.

102.
a. Chronic staphylococcal blepharitis.
b. Other signs:
- mild papillary conjunctivitis
- inferior punctate epitheliopathy
- marginal keratitis
- dry eyes
- styes
- phlyctenulosis (rarely).
c. Treatment:
- regular lid hygiene
- topical antibiotic ointment

- artificial tear substitutes
- weak steroids—when appropriate.
d. Atopic dermatitis.

103.
a. Posterior blepharitis.
b. Classification:
- meibomian seborrhoea
- primary meibomitis
- meibomitis with secondary blepharitis.
c. Treatment:
- systemic antibiotics—tetracycline, doxycycline, or erythromycin
- warm compresses
- artificial tear substitutes
- topical steroids, when appropriate.
d. Systemic associations:
- acne rosacea
- seborrhoeic dermatitis.

104.
a. The upper eyelid and lateral canthus drain into the preauricular nodes and the lower eyelid and medial canthus into the submandibular nodes.
b. Lesions predisposing to squamous cell carcinoma:
- actinic keratosis
- Bowen's disease
- xeroderma pigmentosa
- irradiation.
c. Malignant eyelid tumours:
- basal cell carcinoma
- squamous cell carcinoma
- sebaceous gland carcinoma
- malignant melanoma
- Merkel cell tumour
- Kaposi's sarcoma.

105.
a. Molluscum contagiosum.
b. The causative agent is one of the pox viruses.
c. Chronic follicular conjunctivitis.
d. The lesions are destroyed by expression, cauterization, shave excision or cryotherapy.
e. Corneal micropannus.

106.
a. The main indications are intractable seconary glaucomas which have either failed or are very likely to fail with conventional filtering procedures.
b. Currently used shunts:
- Molteno tube
- Schocket tube and gutter (shown here)

- White pump shunt
- Krupin–Denver valve.
  - c. Complications:
    - blockage of shunt by blood or fibrovascular tissue
    - overdrainage
    - corneal endothelial damage
    - implant erosion.

107.
a. The tumour may originate from:
- meibomian glands
- glands of Zeis
- sebaceous glands in caruncle
- eyebrow.
  - b. Clinical types:
    - Nodular (as shown here)—may masquerade as a 'chalazion'.
    - Spreading—may masquerade as 'chronic blepharitis'.
  - c. Pagetoid spread is extension of the tumour within the epithelium of the conjunctiva.
  - d. Her prognosis is poor because:
    - The upper eyelid is involved.
    - There is maximal diameter of over 10 mm.
    - Duration is over 6 months.

108.
a. Clinical signs:
- moderate to severe bilateral ptosis
- absent upper lid crease
- very deep upper sulci
- entropion of both lower eyelids.
  - b. Involutional aponeurotic ptosis.
  - c. Other types of ptosis in this age group:
    - myogenic, e.g. myasthenia gravis
    - neurogenic, e.g. Horner's syndrome
    - mechanical, e.g. plexiforn neurofibroma
  - d. Operations:
    - levator resection
    - Fasanella–Servat procedure
    - brow suspension
    - aponeurosis strengthening.

109.
a. Main clinical types:
- ocular
- relapsing
- progressive.
  - b. Investigations:
    - Tensilon test—may be combined with a Hess test
    - electromyography to confirm fatigue

- antibodies to acetylcholine receptors and striated muscle
- CT or MR of the anterior mediastinum to rule out thymoma.
c. Other systemic casues of ptosis:
  - myotonic dystrophy
  - ocular myopathies
    - (i) primary
    - (ii) oculopharyngeal
    - (iii) Kearns–Sayre syndrome.

110.
a. There is a fleshy lesion with increased capillarity on the superior bulbar conjunctiva.
b. Differential diagnosis:
  - conjunctival lymphoma—most likely because of the characteristic salmon-patch appearance
  - conjunctival intraepithelial neoplasia (Bowen's disease)
  - invasive squamous cell carcinoma
  - pagetoid spread of a sebaceous gland carcinoma.
c. Biopsy.

111.
a. Severe papillary (cobblestone) conjunctivitis involving the upper tarsus associated with a strand of mucus.
b. Vernal keratoconjunctivitis.
c. About 75% of patients have associated atopy and 66% have a close family history of atopy.
d. Corneal complications:
  - superior punctate epitheliopathy
  - epithelial macroerosions
  - plaque
  - subepithelial scarring
  - pseudogerontoxon.

112.
a. Adenoviruses types 8 and 19.
b. 80% of patients with conjunctivitis.
c. Sequence of corneal changes:
  - Diffuse punctate epithelial keratitis—may clear within 2 weeks.
  - Focal white subepithelial keratitis.
  - Anterior stromal infiltrates—may persist for months.
d. Steroids are indicated for anterior stromal infiltrates impairing visual acuity.

113.
a. Herbert's pits.
b. They are limbal depressions due to cicatrization of follicles and are pathognomonic of trachoma.
c. Grading of trachoma:
  TF = trachomatous follicular inflammation
  TI = trachomatous intense inflammation

TS = trachomatous conjunctival scarring
TT = trachomatous trichiasis
CO = corneal opacity.
d. Other chlamydial infections:
  • adult inclusion conjunctivitis
  • ophthalmia neonatorum.

114.
a. There is extensive subretinal yellowish exudate associated with overlying vascular anomalies.
b. The condition is not hereditary.
c. During the first decade with unilateral:
  • visual loss
  • strabismus
  • leukocoria.
d. Other retinal telangiectasias:
  • idiopathic juxtafoveolar telangiectasis
  • Leber's miliary aneurysms.

115.
a. Reis–Bücklers' corneal dystrophy.
b. Autosomal dominant.
c. There is no associated enzyme defect.
d. The long-term prognosis is reasonably good altough some patients eventually require either lamellar or penetrating keratoplasty. Recurrence of the dystrophy on the graft is common.

116.
a. A conjunctival pseudomembrane consisting of coagulated exudate adherent to inflamed conjunctival epithelium.
b. Causes:
  • adenoviral conjunctivitis
  • vernal disease
  • ligneous conjunctivitis
  • gonococcal conjucnctivitis
  • ocular cicatricial pemphigoid
  • Stevens–Johnson syndrome.
c. A true conjunctival membrane forms when there is necrosis of the conjunctival epithelium and the formation of a fibrovascular adhesion between the conjunctival stroma and the coagulum. Attempted peeling leaves a raw bleeding area. Causes are β-haemolytic streptococcus and diphtheria.

117.
a. Granular corneal dystrophy type 1.
b. Autosomal dominant.
c. There are no systemic associations.
d. Staining is bringt red with Masson trichrome.
e. Between 6/12 and 6/60.

118.
a. Two types:
  - limited form—unilateral affecting the elderly
  - progressive type—bilateal affecting the young.
b. Treatment:
  - topical steroids
  - systemic immunosuppressive agents
  - conjunctival excision in resistant cases.
c. Systemic disease:
  - acne rosacea
  - rheumatoid arthritis
  - systemic lupus erythematosus
  - Wegener's granulomatosis
  - polyarteritis nodosa.

119.
a. Defective depression of the right eye.
b. Right third nerve palsy.
c. Common causes:
  - vascular—pupil usually spared
  - posterior communicating aneurysm—pupil usually involved
  - idiopathic
  - trauma.
d. Uncommon causes:
  - tumours
  - vasculitis associated with collagen vascular disorders
  - syphilis.

120.
a. Sturge–Weber syndrome.
b. The condition is not hereditary.
c. Mechanism of glaucoma:
  - congenital angle anomaly
  - raised episcleral venous pressure due to an episcleral haemangioma.
d. Other ocular lesions:
  - diffuse choroidal haemangioma
  - heterochromia iridis
  - haemangiomas of the iris and ciliary body.

121.
a. Coronal plane.
b. There is a fracture of the medial wall of the left orbit with soft tissue and/or blood in the left ethmoid sinus.
c. Patients with a medial orbital wall fracture often present one or two days after trauma when they blow their nose and the periorbital soft tissue fills with air.
d. The management is:
  - examination of the globe to exclude any ocular damage

- examination of extraocular movements to exclude medial rectus entrapment
- a 10-day course of oral antibiotics
- if there is evidence of air in the soft tissues surrounding the eye the patient is advised to avoid blowing his nose.

122.
a. Axial plane.
b. There is an enlarged left medial recuts muscle.
c. Yes; this explains her diplopia and decreased vision (if the muscle is compressing the optic nerve at the orbital apex).
d. Thyroid-related eye disease; the patient should have thyroid function tests including autoantibodies.

123.
a. Since ocular examination was not possible, the diagnosis is orbital cellulitis until proved otherwise.
b. Cavernous sinus thrombosis.
c. The management here is:
  - Admit the patient.
  - Start intravenous benzylpenicillin, flucloxacillin and metronidazole.
  - Perform a CT scan of the orbitis, brain and sinuses.
  - In cases where ocular examination is possible, extraocular movements, pupil reactions, colour vision and fundoscopy are used to exclude orbital involvement.
  - If at any stage there is suspicion of cavernous sinus thrombosis (sudden onset proptosis which may be bilateral), urgent neurosurgical intervention is needed.

124.
a. Sagittal plane.
b. T1 and T2 refer to two methods of measuring the relaxation times of the excited protons after the magnetic field is switched off. Different tissues have different relaxation times and a certain tissue may be T1 or T2 weighted, implying that it is best visualized on a T1 and T2 image. For normal anatomy T1 weighted images are better while pathological findings are usually better seen on T2 weighted images.
c. This is a T1 weighted image.
d. There is an enlarged mass in the region of the pituitary fossa, most likely a pituitary adenoma.

125.
a. There is a dome-shaped vascular bleb which is consistent with an encapsulated bleb or a tenon's cyst.
b. A cyst-like space has formed from Tenon's capsule over the filtering bleb and this is trapping aqueous. As it enlarges it prevents aqueous from entering the subconjunctival space causing the intraocular pressure to rise.

   c. Treatment options are:
- using aqueous suppressants to prevent the cyst getting any bigger
- regular ocular massage and topical steroid drops
- needling the cyst
- surgical revision of the trabeculectomy
- a combination of the above.

126.
a. A circinate hard exudate.
b. If this circinate was *nasal* to the disc you would just observe. If it were *temporal* to the disc and within the arcades, you would consider focal laser treatment. Remember that hard exudates may resorbe spontaneously but, if they lie near the macula, they may cause maculopathy and a decrease in vision.
c. There is an easy way to remember these by the mnemonic **HAVOX:**

    Haemorrhages—'dot and blot' and flame-shaped
    Aneurysms
    Venous dilatation
    Oedema of the retina due to 'leaky' vessels
    e**X**udates, hard.

127.
a. A large frond of new vessels at the disc.
b. HLA DR3 and DR4.
c. • Vitreous or preretinal haemorrhage.
    • New vessels.
    • Location of new vessels on or near the disc.
    • Severity of new vessels.
d. Panretinal photocoagulation.

128.
a. Arteriovenous nipping.
b. A thickening of the arteriole vessel wall as a result of intimal hyalinization, medial hypertrophy and endothelial hyperplasia. The two causes are age-related (involutional) and hypertension.
c. Grade I—mild generalized arteriolar narrowing
    Grade II—severe narrowing and focal narrowing of arterioles
    Grade III—grade II plus haemorrhages, cotton-wool spots and exudates
    Grade IV—grade III plus disc swelling.

129.
a. Grade 4.
b. Malignant hypertension.
c. Other fundus changes:
- retinal vein occlusion
- retinal artery occlusion

- slow-flow retinopathy due to carotid disease
- anterior ischaemic optic neuropathy
- retinal artery macroaneurysm
- ischaemic choroidal infarcts
- adverse effects on diabetic retinopathy.
  d. Indirect effects:
    - vascular cranial nerve palsies
    - homonymous hemianopia due to CVA.

130.
a. Retinal branch vein occlusion.
b. • Secondary neovascularization which can lead to vitreous haemorrhage
   • Chronic macular oedema.
c. The location of the occlusion is usually at an arteriovenous crossing; there appears to be a common adventitia at these points which allows the artery to impinge on the vein and cause thrombosis under certain circumstances, i.e. arterial disease most commonly secondary to systemic hypertension, diabetes mellitus and age-related arteriosclerosis.

131.
a. Bilateral ectropion.
b. The eyes are watering because the lower lid margin is rolled ·away from the globe so that the inferior puncta are not in apposition to the tear film.
c. Ectropion may be congenital or acquired.
   • Acquired causes are:
       (i)   involutional—due to age-related atrophy
       (ii) neuroparalytic—due to a facial nerve palsy
       (iii) cicatricial—due to trauma, tumours or burns.
   • Congenital causes are rare and may be associated with the blepharophimosis syndrome.

132.
a. Ocular toxocara granuloma.
b. When toxocariasis presents as a systemic infection it is called visceral larva migrans characterized by pyrexia, jaundice, hepatosplenomegaly, pneumonia and occasionally convulsions.
c. The two other common modes of ocular presentation are endophthalmitis and a peripheral granuloma. Other unusual presentations are anterior uveitis with hypopyon, papillitis and vitreous abscess.

133.
a. An old chorioretinal scar adjacent to active chorioretinitis ('satellite' lesion). This is probably an active recurrence of congenital toxoplasmosis.
b. The blurred vision may be explained by vitreous cells and haze caused by the active retinochoroiditis. This inflammation has probably also spilled into the anterior chamber and

caused an anterior uveitis which would explain the photophobia.

c. Yes; at times of decreased immunity it is thought that parasitic cysts rupture, releasing proliferating active parasites that destroy tissue and induce an immune reaction.

134.

a. A chorioretinal scar probably caused by congenital toxoplasmosis.

b. The cat.

c. Congenital toxoplasmosis may be active or inactive at birth. If it is active the two main features are hydrocephalus and necrotizing encephalitis. The latter leads to cerebral calcification, convulsions, jaundice, microcephaly and microphthalmos. The only sign of inactive congenital toxoplasmosis may be chorioretinal scars in the fundus.

135.

a. Infantile esotropia is characterized by the following:
   • a fairly large and stable angle of squint
   • alternating fixation in the primary position and cross fixation on side gaze
   • normal refractive error for the age of the child
   • nystagmus in some cases.

b. Management is as follows:
   • cycloplegic refraction and fundoscopy
   • treatment of amblyopia which occasionally may be present
   • surgery at about the age of 12 months.

c. Potential long-term problems are:
   • undercorrection requiring further surgery
   • inferior oblique overaction
   • dissociated vertical deviation
   • accommodative element requiring spectacle correction amblyopia.

136.

a. Birdshot retinochoroidopathy.

b. There is no underlying metabolic defect.

c. The main vision-threatening complications are:
   • cystoid macular oedema
   • retinal neovascularization and vitreous haemorrhage
   • retinal atrophy
   • optic atrophy.

d. Treatment is with periocular or systemic steroids.

137.

a. Retinal oedema is recognized clinically as thickening of the retina which obscures visualization of the underlying retinal pigment epithelium and choroid.

b. Macular oedema is defined as retinal thickening or hard

exudates within one disc diameter (1500 μm) of the centre of the fovea.

c. Clinically significant macular oedema is defined as:
- retinal thickening within 500 μm of the centre of the fovea
- hard exudates within 500 μm of the centre of the fovea if associated with adjacent retinal thickening (which may be outside the 500 μm limit)
- retinal oedema 1 disc area (1500 μm) or larger, any part of which is within 1 disc diameter of the centre of the fovea.

138.
a. There is a very large subhyaloid haemorrhage overlying the posterior pole as well as several flame-shaped haemorrhages.
b. Strict diabetic control may delay the onset of but will not prevent retinopathy. In some patients aggressive efforts to normalize blood glucose levels with insulin pumps may worsen the retinopathy during the first few months of treatment.
c. Adverse factors are:
- systemic hypertension
- pregnancy
- renal disease
- anaemia.

139.
a. There is severe fibrovascular proliferation with an inferior extramacular tractional retinal detachment.
b. The aims of vitrectomy are:
- restoration of vision by removing vitreous haemorrhage
- prevention of future fibrovascular proliferation by excising vitreous gel
- repair of retinal detachment by excising anteroposterior and bridging tractional membranes.
c. The main indications for vitrectomy are:
- dense persistent vitreous haemorrhage
- dense persistent premacular subhyaloid haemorrhage
- tractional retinal detachment threatening or involving the macula
- combined tractional and rhegmatogenous retinal detachment
- severe and relentlessly progressive fibrovascular proliferation.

140.
a. Melanocytoma of the optic nerve head.
b. Some melanocytomas grow very slowly.
c. The lesion is benign.

   d. Some deep-seated tumours may cause visual impairment by compressing the nerve fibres and their blood supply.

   e. There is no treatment.

141.
a. Ocular reticulum cell sarcoma characterized by vitritis and multifocal subretinal infiltrates.

b. Involvement of the central nervous system by the tumour.

c. Both eyes are eventually affected in 80% of cases.

d. Treatment of the eyes and central nervous system is with radiotherapy.

142.
a. Breast.

b. Bronchus.

c. Prostate.

d. Treatment is palliative with chemotherapy in conjunction with external beam radiotherapy.

e. Other choroidal tumours:
- choroidal naevus
- circumscribed choroidal haemangioma
- diffuse choroidal haemangioma—in Sturge–Weber syndrome
- osteoma
- reticulum cell sarcoma.

143.
a. Other presentations:
- pressure on the lens—displacement, astigmatism and cataract
- extension through the iris root
- posterior extension—retinal detachment
- anterior uveitis due to necrosis
- diffuse circumferential growth—poor prognosis due to late diagnosis.

b. Tests:
- gonioscopy
- transillumination
- ultrasonography
- incision wedge biopsy—in atypical cases.

c. Other tumours:
- medulloepithelioma
- haemangioma
- leiomyoma
- cystic adenoma of pigmented ciliary epithelium.

144.
a. Treatment options:
- nil; if only eye in elderly patient
- enucleation
- radioactive plaque therapy
- cyclotron generated charged particle irradiation
- photocoagulation—only if small

- partial lamellar sclerouveectomy in selected cases
- exenteration, if extrascleral extension
- palliative therapy, if distant metastases.
  b. Adverse factors. Remember the mnemonic SPECS-BAD as follows:
- size—large
- pigmentation
- extrascleral extension
- cell type—epithelioid
- site—anterior to equator
- Bruch's membrane broken
- age—over 65 years
- diffuse growth.

145. a. Three types:
- melanoma arising from primary acquired melanosis
- primary melanoma
- melanoma arising from a pre-existing naevus—very rare.
  b. Overall mortality is 25%.
  c. Tumours arising from the palpebral conjunctiva—50% mortality rate.
  d. Treatment:
- local surgical excision
- exenteration, if spread to the lids
- palliation for metastatic spread.

146. a. Subepithelial.
  b. There is no risk of malignant transformation.
  c. Other lesions:
- hyperpigmentation of facial skin and mucus membranes (naevus of Ota is very common)
- hyperpigmentation of ipsilateral uveal tract (common)
- hyperpigmentation of the trabecular meshwork and glaucoma (uncommon)
- hyperpigmentation of the cornea, lens and optic nerve (rare)
- malignant melanomas of the uvea, skin, orbit and CNS (rare)
- hyperpigmentation of orbit, meninges and brain (very rare).

147. a. Clinical features suggestive of malignancy:
- presence of symptoms
- evidence of growth
- surface lipofuscin pigment
- subretinal fluid
- overlying retina showing cystoid changes

- dilated vessels within the tumour
- location of posterior margin within 3 mm of the optic disc.
  b. Special investigations:
    - ultrasonography to measure thickness
    - fluorescein angiography
    - serial photography.

148. a. Classification:
- Infantile
- Accommodative
    - (i)   refractive
    - (ii) non-refractive
    - (iii) mixed.
- Non-accommodative
    - (i)   stress-induced
    - (ii) sensory deprivation
    - (iii) consecutive
    - (iv) spasm of near reflex
    - (v)   sixth nerve palsy.
  b. Types of amblyopia:
    - strabismic
    - anisometropic—different refractive errors
    - isoametropic—equal large refractive errors
    - sensory deprivation.
  c. Amblyopia therapy:
    - occlusion
    - atropinization
    - manipulation of spectacles
    - pleoptics.

149. a. The vertical cup:disc ratio is 0.9. (The cup is the pale area within the total disc diameter which is devoid of any neural disc tissue). The normal ratio is 0.3–0.5.
  b. One million nerve fibres.
  c. • Systemic conditions:
       –increasing age
       –diabetes
       –hypertension
       –systemic vascular disease.
     • Ocular conditions:
       –myopia
       –Fuchs' endothelial dystrophy
       –retinitis pigmentosa.
  d. The diagnosis of primary open angle glaucoma depends on the following:
    - normal anterior chamber angles

- raised intraocular pressures
- pathologically cupped discs
- visual field loss.

Given the fact that there is raised intraocular pressure with the above appearance of the disc, the diagnosis of primary open-angle glaucoma can be made, though ideally documented field loss should be present.

150.
a. Retinal artery macroaneurysm.
b. Causes of visual loss:
  - retinal haemorrhage
  - retinal oedema
  - hard exudate formation
  - retinal branch vein occlusion
  - vitreous haemorrhage.
c. Early laser treatment of macular oedema and exudation may be beneficial.

151.
a. Peters' anomaly.
b. Autosomal dominant.
c. Other ocular anomalies:
  - Glaucoma—in 50%.
  - Anterior cataract.
  - Miscellaneous uncommon associations:
    - (i) cornea plana
    - (ii) sclerocornea
    - (iii) microphthalmos
    - (iv) corectopia
    - (v) iris hypoplasia.
d. There are no systemic associations.

152.
a. Opacification types:
  - Elschnig's pearls due to proliferation of lens epithelium
  - opacification associated with residual subcapsular plaque
  - capsular fibrosis.
b. Indications for capsulotomy:
  - diminished visual acuity
  - severe glare or monocular diplopia
  - impaired visualization of the fundus for diagnostic or therapeutic purposes.
c. Six months or more after the initial cataract extraction.
d. Potential complications:
  - damage to the implant
  - elevation of intraocular pressure
  - cystoid macular oedema
  - retinal detachment.

153.

a. Lid signs:
- lid retraction in primary gaze—Dalrymple's sign (shown here)
- lid lag in downgaze—von Graefe's sign
- staring and frightened appearance—Kocher's sign
- infrequent blinking
- fine tremor on lid closure
- jerky spasmodic movements on lid opening.

b. Surgical procedures:
- inferior rectus recession
- excision of Müller's muscle
- recession of levator aponeurosis
- recession of lower lid retractors.

c. Other causes:
- Congenital (very rare).
- Neurological
  - (i) Marcus—Gunn jaw-winking
  - (ii) aberrant regeneration of the third nerve
  - (iii) Collier's sign of the dorsal midbrain (Parinaud's syndrome).
- Mechanical
  - (i) post-traumatic
  - (ii) surgical over-correction
  - (iii) unilateral ptosis with contralateral levator overaction.
- Metabolic
  - (i) cirrhosis
  - (ii) uraemia.

154.

a. Other features:
- associated anterior scleritis in 80%
- disc oedema
- vitritis
- choroidal folds
- retinal changes
  - –macular oedema
  - –exudative detachment
  - –subretinal exudation and subretinal mass
  - –intraretinal white deposits.

b. Differential diagnosis:
- choroidal tumour
- orbital inflammatory disease
- uveal effusion syndrome
- Harada's disease.

c. Differences from retinal detachment:
- absence of photopsia and floaters

- frequently very low intraocular pressure—anterior chamber may be shallow
- appearance
  - convex, smooth, immobile, brown elevations
  - does not involve posterior pole
  - peripheral retina and ora serrata easily seen.

155.

a. Foville's syndrome characterized by ipsilateral:
  - sixth nerve palsy combined with gaze palsy
  - facial palsy and analgesia
  - Horner's syndrome
  - diminished hearing.
b. Millard–Gubler syndrome:
  - ipsilateral sixth nerve palsy
  - contralateral hemiplegia
  - variable signs of a dorsal pontine lesion.
c. Basilar lesions:
  - raised intracranial pressure
  - fractures
  - acoustic neuroma
  - nasopharyngeal tumours.

156.

a. Hyperpigmentation:
  - pigment dispersion syndrome
  - pseudoexfoliation syndrome
  - following blunt trauma
  - following acute angle-closure glaucoma
  - anterior uveitis
  - diabetes
  - naevus of Ota.
b. Main types of gonioscopes:
  - Direct—provide direct view of angle
    (i) diagnostic—Koeppe
    (ii) surgical—Swan–Jacob, Barkan, Thorpe etc.
  - Indirect diagnostic—Goldmann, Zeiss.
c. Shaffer grade 2: a moderately narrow angle in which only the trabeculum can be identified.

157.

a. There are fine keratic precipitates scattered throughout the corneal endothelium.
b. Fuchs' heterochromic cyclitis.
c. Other signs:
  - mild aqueous flare and cells
  - iris atrophy and heterochromia
  - Koeppe nodules
  - mild rubeosis iridis
  - absence of posterior synechiae

- mild vitritis
- fine blood vessels in the anterior chamber angle.
d. Management:
   - There is no effective treatment for the uveitis.
   - There is no contraindication to standard cataract surgery.
   - Long-term follow-up is required because of the risk of subsequent development of glaucoma.

158.
a. Drainage complications:
   - choroidal haemorrhage
   - retinal incarceration
   - iatrogenic tear formation
   - vitreous prolapse
   - postoperative endophthalmitis.
b. Early failure:
   - immobile retina due to proliferative vitreoretinopathy
   - buckle failure—inadequate height, inadequate size, incorrect position
   - fishmouthing of break
   - complications of drainage of subretinal fluid
   - missed break.
c. Late failure:
   - proliferative vitreoretinopathy
   - re-opening of break due to inadequate buckle
   - re-opening of break due to insufficient cryotherapy
   - new break formation.

159.
a. Ocular motility is restricted by oedema during the active infiltrative phase and by fibrotic contracture during the fibrotic stage.
b. Motility defects:
   - defective elevation—fibrotic inferior rectus (shown here)
   - defective abduction—fibrotic medial rectus
   - defective depression—fibrotic superior rectus
   - defective adduction—fibrotic lateral rectus.
c. Indications for decompression:
   - cosmetic
   - optic neuropathy unresponsive to other measures
   - exposure keratopathy due to severe proptosis.
d. Types of decompression:
   - two wall—antral-ethmoidal
   - three wall—antral-ethmoidal plus lateral wall
   - four wall—three wall plus part of sphenoid and roof.

160.
a. Treatment:
   - systemic steroids in the first instance.

- immunosuppressive agents (cyclophosphamide, azathioprine, cyclosporin) in steroid-resistant cases
- combined immunosuppressives and pulsed intravenous methylprednisolone as a last resort.

b. Causes:
- rheumatoid arthritis—most common
- Wegener's granulomatosis
- polyarteritis nodosa
- systemic lupus erythematosus
- systemic arteritis
- relapsing polychondritis.

c. Treatment of non-necrotizing scleritis:
- topical steroids for associated episcleritis
- oral fluriprofen or indomethacin
- systemic steroids as last resort.

161.
a. Direct carotid-cavernous fistula.
b. Causes:
- basal skull fracture—most common cause
- intracavernous rupture of an aneurysm or an arteriosclerotic artery.

c. Other signs:
- pulsatile proptosis associated with a bruit abolished by ipsilateral carotid compression
- raised intraocular pressure
- rubeosis iridis
- ophthalmoplegia
- retinal vascular engorgement or central retinal vein occlusion.

d. Dynamic proptosis:
- Pulsatile with a bruit
    (i) carotid-cavernous fistula
    (ii) orbital arteriovenous malformation.
- Pulsatile without a bruit
    (i) congenital defect in sphenoid bone, neurofibromatosis type 1
    (ii) defect in orbital roof
    (iii) indirect carotid-cavernous fistula.
- Intermittent but not pulsatile
    (i) orbital varices
    (ii) orbital capillary haemangioma.

162.
a. Conjunctival phlyctenulosis.
b. A non-specific delayed hypersensitivity reaction to staphylococcal or other bacterial agents.
c. May involve the cornea and cause scarring, ulceration and rarely perforation.

d. Topical steroids and, rarely, systemic tetracycline.
e. Differential diagnosis:
  • nodular episcleritis
  • inflamed pinguecula.

163.
a. Cornea verticillata (vortex dystrophy).
b. Systemic diseases:
  • rheumatoid arthritis or a collagen vascular disease treated with choloroquine
  • gout treated with indomethacin
  • cardiac arrhythmia treated with amiodarone
  • carcinoma of the breast treated with tamoxifen
  • schizophrenia on long-term chlorpromazine
  • Fabry's disease.
c. The following drugs may cause retinal changes:
  • chloroquine—maculopathy
  • tamoxifen—minute, superficial, crystalline ring-like deposits at the macula.

164.
a. Band keratopathy.
b. Chronic anterior uveitis associated with juvenile chronic arthritis.
c. Other causes:
  • idiopathic in the elderly
  • chronic anterior uveitis in adults
  • phthisis bulbi
  • increased serum calcium or phosphorus levels (rare).
d. Treatment:
  • chelation with sodium versenate
  • excimer laser keratectomy.

165.
a. Cafe-au-lait spot.
b. Neurofibromatosis type 1 (NF I).
c. Classification:
  NF-I = von Recklinghausen's disease
  (i) cafe-au-lait spots
  (ii) Lisch nodules
  (iii) neurofibromas
  NF-II = bilateral acoustic neuromas
  NF-III = segmental neurofibromatosis
  NF-IV = multiple cafe-au-lait spots only.
d. Differential diagnosis of congenital iris nodules:
  • Brushfield spots (Trisomy 21)
  • juvenile xanthogranuloma
  • Lisch nodules
  • naevi
  • cysts.

166.
a. Hering's law of equal innervation.
b. There is a *right* lateral rectus palsy. The more restricted chart is that of the eye with the paretic muscle; the restriction will be greatest in the direction of action of the affected muscle. (The chart is labelled as 'field of eye' and 'fixing eye'; the former annotation indicates which eye's muscles are being examined).
c. No; the patient must have normal retinal correspondence for this test to be accurate.

167.
a. There is restriction of upgaze and to a lesser extent downgaze in the left eye.
b. A rule of thumb to differentiate between innervational defects and mechanical ones is to compare the shape of the inner and outer fields: in innervational defects the two are asymmetrically distorted while in mechanical ones the two are unchanged or symmetrically distorted.
c. Left blow out fracture with tethering of the inferior rectus muscle.

168.
a. There is restriction of abduction and upgaze in the left eye with corresponding overactions in the right eye.
b. This is probably a mechanical defect because:
   • Innervational defect would involve a VI nerve palsy with a partial III nerve palsy which is very unlikely
   • The inner and outer fields of the Hess chart are fairly symmetrical.
c. Thyroid-related ophthalmopathy.

169.
a. This is a 'V' pattern deviation.
b. No; inferior oblique palsies are associated with 'A' pattern horizontal deviations.
c. This is the typical 'dog ears' Hess chart seen in Brown's syndrome.
d. Aetiology is:
   • Congenital—abnormality of the superior oblique tendon distal to the trochlear.
   • Acquired
      (i) trochlear inflammation, e.g. rheumatoid arthritis
      (ii) iatrogenic, such as post superior oblique tendon tuck
      (iii) trauma.

170.
a. This means that each point in the visual field is presented with a stimulus known to be brighter than the expected normal value for that point. This is used as a quick screening test; if a stimulus is not seen, a defect is noted but its extent is not determined.

b. Enlarged blind spots.
c. Causes are:
- chronic papilloedema
- high myopia
- myelinated nerve fibres
- optic disc drusen
- glaucoma
- peripapillary choroiditis.

171.
a. There are crystal-like deposits in the cornea.
b. Possible causes are:
- Corneal dystrophy
    (i) Schnyder's crystalline dystrophy
    (ii) Bietti's marginal crystalline dystrophy.
- Metabolic disorders
    (i)   Cystinosis
    (ii) Tyrosinosis
    (iii) Gout
    (iv) Tangier disease
    (v)   LCAT (lecithin-cholesterol acyltransferase) deficiency.
- Haematological disorders
    (i) Multiple myeloma
    (ii) Other monoclonal gammopathies.
- Infection—infectious crystalline keratopathy (most commonly reported with *Staphylococcus aureus* infections).
- Others—secondary lipid keratopathy.

172.
a. There is hyperostosis involving the sphenoid bone on the left side.
b. A similar sign may be seen in:
- sphenoid ridge meningioma—most likely diagnosis in this case
- fibrous dysplasia—patients are usually much younger
- Paget's disease of bone—much more widespread
- osteoma.

173.
a. A child may present because:
- The parents notice
    (i)   leukocoria
    (ii) an opacity 'in the pupil' (usually only if anterior polar cataract and very observant parents)
    (iii) that the child 'does not follow them' with his eyes
    (iv) that the child has a squint

    (v) that the child has photophobia (due to glare with certain cataracts).

  • A paediatrician
    (i) is screening the child for failure to thrive
    (ii) has diagnosed a syndrome which is associated with congenital cataracts.

 b. Aetiology of congenital cataracts is:
  • **I**diopathic
  • **G**enetic
    (i) Simple
    (ii) Chromosomal disorders, e.g. trisomy 18.
  • **I**ntrauterine infection
    (i) Rubella
    (ii) Varicella
    (iii) Toxoplasmosis.
  • **M**etabolic
    (i) With an unwell child, e.g. galactosaemia, Lowe's syndrome, Refsum's disease.
    (ii) With a healthy child, e.g. galactokinase deficiency.
  • Associated with **O**cular anomalies e.g. aniridia, posterior lenticonus, persistent hyperplastic primary vitreous.
  • Associated with **S**ystemic syndromes, e.g. incontinentia pigmenti, congenital ichthyosis.

174.
 a. Frontal bossing/saddle nose/poorly developed maxilla/rhagades (linear scars at the angles of the mouth). Her teeth, if visible, would probably have shown peg-like features (Hutchinson's teeth).
 b. Hutchinson's triad (interstitial keratitis, deafness and Hutchinson's teeth) is suggestive of congenital syphilis.
 c. Ocular manifestations of congenital syphilis:
  • interstitial keratitis (IK)
  • retinopathy, either of a 'salt and pepper' variety or of a type that resembles retinitis pigmentosa
  • optic atrophy
  • corneal opacities (usually scars from old IK).

175.
 a. Chronic papilloedema.
 b. The finding of papilloedema with a normal MR scan is suggestive of idiopathic intracranial hypertension.
 c. Apart from headaches and intracranial noises (which are the commonest) other symptoms include transient visual obscurations, sparkles, visual loss and diplopia (due to sixth nerve palsy).
 d. A lumbar puncture to show raised cerebrospinal fluid opening pressure.

176.
a. This is a left exotropia (manifest divergent squint).
b. There are three types:
- Monocular cover-uncover test: to differentiate between a tropia (manifest) and a phoria (latent) deviation, e.g. if the right eye is covered and then uncovered and the left eye moves there is a tropia; if the right eye moves while it is being uncovered there is a phoria.
- Alternate cover test: measures the total deviation (latent and manifest); the eyes are covered and uncovered quickly and alternately, thereby causing dissociation of the eyes.
- Prism and cover test: measures the amount of deviation in prism dioptres while both eyes are uncovered, e.g. if the right eye is fixing on an object, it is covered while at the same time a prism (appropriately orientated) is placed in front of the left eye; larger prisms are used until there is no movement by the left eye to take up fixation when the fixing right eye is covered.

177.
a. The picture shows leukocoria (white reflex from the left eye); this is retinoblastoma until proven otherwise.
b. The differential diagnosis of leukocoria in a child is a chestnut of a question; if you fail to impress upon the examiner that you know this and understand its implications, you're struggling! Here is one method of remembering the list:
- Conditions that involve the pupil/lens
    (i) congenital cataract
    (ii) cyclitic membrane.
- Conditions that involve the vitreous
    (i) toxocara endophthalmitis (also involves retina)
    (ii) persistent hyperplastic primary vitreous
    (iii) organized vitreous haemorrhage
    (iv) vitreous abscess.
- Conditions that involve the retina
    (i) tumours, e.g. retinoblastoma, retinal astrocytoma
    (ii) retinopathy of prematurity
    (iii) vascular anomalies, e.g. Coats' disease, angiomatosis retinae
    (iv) congenital, e.g. retinal dysplasia, retinochoroidal coloboma, extensive myelinated nerve fibres
    (v) total retinal detachment, e.g. incontinentia pigmenti, Norrie's disease.

178.
a. Retinal astrocytoma.
b. Astrocytic hamartoma of the brain in association with tuberous sclerosis.
c. Autosomal dominant.

d. Skin lesions:
- angiofibromas (adenoma sebaceum)
- ash-leaf hypopigmented patches which fluoresce with ultraviolet light
- skin tags (molluscum fibrosum pendulum)
- forehead fibrous plaques
- shagreen patches.

179.
a. A space-occupying lesion arising from the medial third of the sphenoidal ridge. The diagnosis is a sphenoidal ridge meningioma.
b. No; meningiomas arising from the medial third of the sphenoidal ridge tend to cause visual loss and optic atrophy much earlier than proptosis, in complete contrast to those arising from the middle and lateral thirds.
c. Meningiomas arise from arachnoid cells on the deep surface of the dura and from arachnoid prolongations into the dura.
d. The presence of calcified spheres called psammoma bodies in the centre of whorls of elongated cells seen histologically is suggestive of meningioma.

180.
a. CT scan shows 3 areas of calcification in the frontal areas.
b. The differential diagnosis of the CT scan is:
- cerebral secondaries
- tuberculosis
- toxoplasmosis
- histoplasmosis
- coccidiomycosis
- cryptococcus infection
- candidiasis.
c. In any patient presenting with unusual infections a cause for immunodeficiency must be loooked for; in the elderly this tends to be underlying malignancy while in the young HIV infection must be excluded.

181.
a. Cataracts may be described in terms of aetiology, morphology and maturity.

Aetiology	Morphology	Maturity
• age-related	• nuclear	• immature
• congenital	• cortical	• mature
• metabolic	• lamellar	• intumescent
• traumatic	• capsular	• hypermature
• drug-induced	• subcapsular	• Morgagnian.
• secondary to ocular disease	• sutural	
• associated with systemic syndromes		

b. Morgagnian.
c. • Intracapsular (where the lens and lens capsule are removed)
   • Extracapsular (where the lens capsule is opened and the lens is removed with the remaining capsule left in situ)
   • Phacoemulsification (the same as extracapsular except that the lens is fragmented into an emulsification by a vibrating probe and then aspirated; in extracapsular cataract extraction the lens is expressed whole)
   • Lensectomy (where the whole lens including the capsule is removed using a vitreous cutter either through a limbal or a pars plana approach)
   • Simple aspiration (largely superceded by lensectomy for treatment of infantile cataract).

182.
a. Roth's spot: a white centred haemorrhage.
b. Systemic disease:
   • bacterial endocarditis
   • leukaemia
   • multiple myeloma
   • anaemia
   • rare cases include candidiasis and fungal endophthalmitis.
c. In the hyperviscosity syndromes the viscosity of blood is raised such that it becomes symptomatic. It may be raised due to either increased components of plasma (e.g. protein in multiple myeloma) or increased number of cells (e.g. cells in leukaemia).

183.
a. In the embryo in order to allow the hyaloid vessels to run in the centre of the optic nerve, a fissure forms inferiorly and extends from the front of the eye to half-way along the optic stalk (embryonal equivalent of the optic nerve). The fissure closes by fusion starting in its middle and extending both anteriorly and posteriorly. Failure of fusion leads to colobomas of the disc, retina, choroid and iris.
b. Yes; a typical retinochoroidal coloboma involves the region of the embryonal fissure, i.e. mainly inferonasally.
c. About 60%.

184.
a. Optic disc coloboma without retinochoroidal involvement.
b. Over 50% subsequently develop serous retinal detachment at the macula. Other associations are orbital cysts and retinal dysplasia.
c. The systemic associations are:

- Aicardi syndrome, an inherited disorder limited to females in which there are chorioretinal lesions, optic nerve head coloboma, microphthalmos and agenesis of corpus callosum seen on CT scan; affected patients have severe mental retardation and infantile spasms
- Trisomy 13
- Goldenhar's syndrome (a few reported cases)
- Transphenoidal or transethmoidal basal encephalocoele.

185.

a. • Veins are not dilated.
- Vessels are not obscured as they cross the disc.
- Disc is pink and not hyperaemic.

b. Optic nerve head drusen; also suggested by an anomalous vascular branching pattern and 'lumpy' disc margins.

c. This may be:
- Congenital
  - (i) optic nerve head drusen
  - (ii) hypermetropia.
- Acquired
  - (i) papilloedema (raised intracranial pressure)
    - –space occupying lesion
    - –idiopathic intracranial hypertension
    - –hydrocephalus
  - (ii) tumour
    - –compressing the optic nerve, e.g. meningioma
    - –rarely, metastases infiltrating optic nerve head
  - (iii) inflammation
    - –papillitis
    - –uveitis, e.g. sarcoid and rarely acute anterior uveitis
  - (iv) vascular disorders
    - –anterior ischaemic optic neuropathy
    - –central retinal vein occlusion
  - (v) marked ocular hypotony, e.g. post surgery
  - (vi) malignant hypertension
  - (vii) Leber's hereditary optic neuropathy.

186.

a. Congenital optic disc pit with mild retinal epithelial changes at the macula.

b. Serous detachment of the macula.

c. The subretinal fluid is thought to be derived from one of the following:
- vitreous
- cerebrospinal fluid
- leaking vessels from within the pit.

d. 10% of optic pits are bilateral.

187.
a. This is because a paramagnetic substance called gadolinium DTPA (diethylenetriaminepenta-acetic acid) has been used as contrast. This is taken up by tumour circulation and appears bright white on T1 weighted MR scans. In this case the tumour is likely to be a pituitary adenoma.

b. A junctional scotoma—as exquisite a pointer of pituitary tumours as bilateral superotemporal hemianopias.

c. The main difference between MR and CT scan is that the former relies on a pulse of electromagnetic waves (generated by activating a strong magnetic field) which excite protons (hydrogen ions) which then re-emit the energy gained as they relax (i.e. when the magnetic field is switched off). This signal is recorded in terms of location and intensity. In CT scanning X-rays are used (i.e. ionizing radiation) and the relative rates of tissue absorption recorded.

188.
a. There are white nodular lesions on the iris that become confluent in areas.

b. With this history infiltrating retinoblastoma must be excluded. Other causes may be:
- leukaemia
- amelanotic melanoma
- a granulomatous uveitis.

c. Retinoblastoma may be hereditary or non-hereditary. 20% of patients with a deletion of 13q develop retinoblastoma. The normal allele probably regulates proliferation and its absence probably leads to uncontrolled proliferation.
Two steps are necessary to induce malignancy:
- The first occurs in a single somatic retinal cell (non-hereditary) or in a germ line cell (hereditary).
- In both hereditary and non-hereditary tumours the second step is a somatic event in a retinal cell that then becomes malignant.

189.
a. Optic atrophy.

b. Causes of bilateral, acquired optic atrophy:
- glaucoma
- drugs such as ethambutol, streptomycin, isoniazid, antabuse, heavy metals, chlorpropramide, chloramphenicol, digitalis and vincristine
- toxic deficiency state, vitamin B_{12} and thiamine deficiency (tobacco-alcohol amblyopia)
- post chronic papilloedema
- demyelination
- systemic syndromes such as mucopolysaccharidoses, leukodystrophies, Conradi's syndrome.

c. Causes of unilateral optic atrophy:

- glaucoma
- inflammatory—optic/retrobulbar neuritis (idiopathic or due to multiple sclerosis)
- vascular
    - (i) anterior or posterior ischaemic optic neuropathy
    - (ii) post central retinal artery occlusion
- tumour
    - (i) compressing the optic nerve, e.g. orbital or parasellar tumours
    - (ii) intrinsic optic nerve tumour, e.g. glioma
    - (iii) infiltrative lesions, e.g. lymphoma
- endocrine—thyroid eye disease with enlarged muscles compressing the optic nerve
- trauma—optic nerve transection
- post chronic papilloedema.

190.

a. Ammonia is a powerful alkali which can saponify lipids in the corneal epithelium and bind the collagen and mucopolysaccharides of the corneal and conjunctival stroma. This causes perilimbal ischaemia with two main consequences:
- damage to limbal stem cells that are responsible for replenishing corneal epithelium
- formation of fibrovascular tissue which invades the damaged cornea (pannus). Damage to associated conjunctiva and lids causes adhesions to form with obliteration of the fornices.

b.
- 500–1000 ml normal saline irrigation of the affected eyes.
- Assess the degree of perilimbal ischaemia and size of epithelial defect.
- Start topical antibiotic, steroid and potassium ascorbate drops together with oral ascorbic acid. Patient may have to be admitted if severe injury.

191.

a. This is a spontaneous hyphaema (blood in the anterior chamber).

b. Causes of spontaneous hyphaema are all acquired.
- Tumour
    - (i) intraocular neoplasms such as retinoblastoma
    - (ii) juvenile xanthogranuloma.
- Inflammation, e.g. severe iritis.
- Infection
    - (i) herpes simplex keratouveitis
    - (ii) herpes zoster iritis.
- Haematological disorders
    - (i) leukaemia
    - (ii) haemophilia.
- Vascular disorders, e.g. rubeosis iridis.

192.
a. Corneal reflex.
b. In any patient with sensorineural deafness and facial weakness it is important to be concerned about the possibility of a cerebellopontine angle tumour, especially an acoustic neuroma. In these cases absence of the corneal reflex increases the suspicion of such a tumour.
c. A CT or MR scan should be performed.

193.
a. Bullous keratopathy.
b. Endothelial decompensation.
c. Following cataract surgery and implantation of an anterior chamber intraocular lens.
d. Other causes:
  • Fuchs' endothelial dystrophy
  • post-traumatic
  • post-inflammatory.
e. Treatment options:
  • hypertonic saline and frequent use of lubricants
  • soft bandage contact lenses
  • penetrating keratoplasty.

194.
a. Causes of shallow orbits are:
  • craniostenoses, e.g. Crouzon's disease and Apert's syndrome
  • chromosomal abnormalities, e.g. trisomy 18 and trisomy 13–15
  • rare conditions, e.g. osteogenesis imperfecta, hypophosphataemia.
b. Other causes of bilateral proptosis in a child are:
  • haematological
    (i) leukaemia
    (ii) lymphoma
  • neoplastic
    (i) metastatic neuroblastoma
    (ii) histiocytosis X
    (iii) sinus histiocytosis
  • inflammatory
    (i) Wegener's granulomatosis
    (ii) orbital myositis
  • vascular—cavernous sinus thrombosis.

195.
a. Because there is active retinochoroiditis, inflammatory cells have spilled into the overlying vitreous making it hazy.
b. Toxoplasmosis or candidiasis. In patients with AIDS, other opportunistic infections must also be considered, e.g. early cytomegalovirus retinitis or tuberculosis.
c. The dye test is based on the fact that living organisms

exposed to normal serum take up methylene blue but not if serum (undiluted) has anti-toxoplasma IgG.

d. Specific IgG detectable by dye test persists for many years following exposure to toxoplasma, whether acquired in utero or during the post natal period. The significance of the dye test depends on rising titres. Titres of 1 : 64 may persist for years.

196.
a. Unlikely because bony breast secondaries are usually lytic and not opaque as is this lesion.

b. The edge of the lesion is very smooth suggesting an air–tissue interface. The lesion is probably in the frontal sinus and could be a mucocele. If it were outside the sinus it could be a dermoid.

c. Orbital bony metastases:
- breast
- bronchus
- prostate
- skin melanoma
- kidney
- gastrointestinal tract.

197.
a. Background, pre-proliferative and proliferative. Added to these is maculopathy which may accompany any of the three. Some also add end-stage disease as the fifth type.

b. The type shown in pre-proliferative. There are five features to this, easily remembered by the mnemonic **CIVAL**:
- **C**otton-wool spots
- **I**rma—intraretinal microvascular abnormalities
- **V**enous changes—beading/looping/sausage-like segmentation
- **A**rteriolar narrowing
- **L**arge dark blot haemorrhages.

Also in the above case there may be an element of macular oedema (not readily apparent on photographs) which would explain the impaired vision.

c. Pre-proliferative retinopathy does not warrant panretinal photocoagulation but does demand frequent fundoscopy (e.g. 3–4 monthly). Whether the macula is ischaemic or oedematous can be determined using fluorescein angiography.

198.
a. Bilateral hilar lymphadenopathy.
b. Sarcoidosis.
c. Eyelid lesions:
- lupus pernio—violaceous plaques

- granulomas of the lid margin—mistaken for chalazia
- various infiltrative lesions.
  d. Anterior segment lesions:
  - granulomas of conjunctiva, episclera and, rarely, sclera
  - keratoconjunctivitis sicca
  - acute anterior uveitis—usually acute in young patients with hilar adenopathy
  - chronic anterior uveitis—usually in older patients with lung fibrosis.

199. a. Hard exudates typically form peripheral to chronic vascular leakage either from abnormal retinal or choroidal blood vessels.
b. Classification:
  - Retinal vascular leakage
    - (i) diabetic retinopathy
    - (ii) old retinal vein occlusion
    - (iii) hypertensive retinopathy
    - (iv) retinal artery macroaneurysm
    - (v) retinal telangiectasias
    - (vi) papilloedema.
  - Subretinal vascular leakage
    - (i) choroidal neovascular membranes
    - (ii) choroidal tumours.

200. a. Neovascular maculopathy due to subretinal choroidal neovascularization.
b. HLA-B7—associated with maculopathy.
c. The vitreous is always normal in this condition.
d. Causes of multifocal inflammation:
  - acute posterior placoid pigment epitheliopathy
  - sympathetic uveitis
  - syphilis
  - multifocal choroiditis and panuveitis
  - punctate inner choroidopathy
  - birdshot retinochoroidopathy
  - multiple evanescent white-dot syndrome (MEWS)
  - toxoplasma punctate retinitis.

Index

Note: entries are indexed **by question numbers** and matching answers.